GAY
SEX
GAY
HEALTH

GAY SEX, GAY HEALTH

All you need to know about gay sex and sexual health

DR ALEX VASS

Vermilion
LONDON

1 3 5 7 9 10 8 6 4 2

First published in the United Kingdom in 2006 by Vermilion
an imprint of Ebury Publishing
Random House UK Ltd
Random House
20 Vauxhall Bridge Road
London SW1V 2SA

Random House Australia (Pty) Limited
20 Alfred Street, Milsons Point, Sydney
New South Wales 2061, Australia

Random House New Zealand Limited
18 Poland Road, Glenfield
Auckland 10, New Zealand

Random House (Pty) Limited
Isle of Houghton Corner Boundary Road & Carse O'Gowrie
Houghton 2198, South Africa

Random House Publishers India Private Limited
301 World Trade Tower, Hotel Intercontinental Grand Complex
Barakhamba Lane, New Delhi 110 001, India

Random House UK Limited Reg. No. 954009
www.randomhouse.co.uk
Papers used by Vermilion are natural, recyclable products
made from wood grown in sustainable forests.

A CIP catalogue record is available for this book from the British Library.

ISBN: 0091912628
ISBN 13: 9780091912628 (from January 2007)

Interior designed by seagulls.net

Printed and bound in Great Britain by Clays Ltd, Elcograf S.p.A.

Penguin Random House is committed to a sustainable future for
our business, our readers and our planet. This book is made from
Forest Stewardship Council® certified paper.

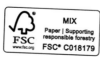

ACKNOWLEDGEMENTS

Firstly to all the men who shared their stories, questions and concerns – they were the inspiration for this book. Next to a number of people who provided their time and expertise in commenting on and so improving this book. Tim Foskett (PACE) and Ford Hickson (Sigma) for the Gay Life section, Barrie Dwyer (GMFA) for help with the Sex section, Dr Martin Hourihan and Dr Alan McOwan for looking over the medical content, especially the Sex Problems section, Johnathan Finney (Stonewall) for legal advice, Grainne Whalley (Antidote) and Dr Matthew Shields for reading through the Drugs section and John Beveridge for advice over sex addiction. Special thanks to Will Nutland (Terrence Higgins Trust) and David Hudson (*Boyz* magazine) for reading through the whole thing.

Thanks also to Gavin for passing me the Boyzdoc column that started this all off, my editor Julia Kellaway for making it all happen, and to friends and sisters for their ideas and enthusiasm.

INTRODUCTION

Who needs a book about gay sex and health? You may be a guy who already knows a fair bit about the subject because you've been having sex with men for a while, or maybe you're just starting out and it all seems to be happening quite naturally and nicely, thank you! Whatever stage you're at, this book can offer you some tips on how to have better, more fulfilling sex, while safeguarding your health. We spend so much of our lives learning about other things or training ourselves to look good that I promise you that a little time spent reading about sex and your health will pay dividends and lead you towards a healthier and more enjoyable sex life.

Sex between men is something to celebrate and something to cultivate. However, while many men feel confident in what they do, just as many can feel unsure about whether they are doing it right. Many, too, have questions about how their health can be affected through sex or want to know what the problem might be when things aren't quite right with their body. Most men know that in sex, as with many aspects of life, along with the pleasures can go potential problems, risks or dangers, like sexually transmitted infections.

Every part of your body that you use for sex has its own set of health problems that can crop up from time to time. Sex can also bring up a range of emotional and psychological issues that can result in sexual problems such as impotence (erectile dysfunction). So learning a bit more about sex, physical,

CONTENTS

PART IV: SEX PROBLEMS

PART V: DRUGS

mental and emotional health, and how they all interact, will help you to spot, and deal with, potential problems early on. Prompt detection often makes them easier to sort out.

Gay sex education is not widely available, and so a lot of what we learn about comes either from just doing it, or from sources that can give a distorted view of what gay sex is all about, such as porn films, magazines – and even friends! So I hope that this book can help a little to dispel some myths about gay sex. For example, gay men can have a reputation for being 'up for' sex all the time and for having lots of it. Although this is often not the case, it can still make some gay men feel that they need to live up to this reputation. Many gay men do enjoy a varied and full sex life and find it easy to find sex. But that is not everyone's experience. No two gay men are the same – some prefer having sex with many different partners while others prefer a long-term monogamous relationship. Some guys like lots of different types of sex while others prefer to keep within a narrow spectrum of activities. Part III of this book will show you that gay men can be very varied in where, how often and what kind of sex they enjoy.

Many guys want to know how to have great sex. Knowledge, about your body, about how it works, and about what can go wrong, is the first step. This can give you new confidence about why you feel the way you do, and so lead you toward a more fulfilling sex life. There is, therefore, a section in this book all about the parts of the body you use for sex. Technique and practice are also important. And so this book covers most sex acts and gives some tips that may help you to do what you enjoy better and with more confidence – while offering advice on any health risks involved.

Great sex is also about feeling free within yourself and allowing yourself to use your imagination. We still live in a world where being gay is not universally accepted. And most men, myself included, have had to go through difficult stages in coming to terms with their sexuality. Feeling bad about who you are will affect your sexual life and the choices you make. Sex is the act that ultimately defines your sexuality and so it is tied up with who you are and how you feel about yourself. It is often central to emotional relationships, too. So I believe that the more confident you become with who you are and what you like doing, the better able you will be to express, and nurture, your sexuality. Ultimately, this will help you to have a more satisfying emotional and sexual life. That's why this book covers topics such as being gay, coming out and some of the issues around boyfriends and relationships.

All the personal stories in this book are here to illustrate that there are men like you who have questions about sex, their sexuality and about their health. So you will see that whatever your problem or worry, you are not alone. The comments printed in this book have come from guys writing to me at *Boyz* magazine, from personal experience, and from the men I talk to. Their comments have been paraphrased and names have been changed – not through embarrassment, but because it allowed them to be more honest about their experiences.

Now a note about the word 'gay'. I've used it a lot in this book. What you like to call yourself is up to you. This book is for any man who has sex with other men – whether he sees himself as 'gay', 'bisexual', 'straight' or just happens to like to having sex with men now and then.

Finally, you might ask, who am I to write about sex, relationships and sexual health? Well, as a GP I know a bit about the body and what can go wrong with it. But I've also had sex – both good, bad and great – and, being gay, I've been through many of the experiences and difficulties that this book covers. Where I haven't, I've read and listened to what others had to say. I wish I'd known everything here when I was starting out. Writing it has certainly taught me a thing or two! If you find some of the information useful or just interesting then it will have made writing the book worthwhile. So, good luck to you all and happy reading!

PART I
GAY
LIFE

ONE

BEING GAY

'It took me a long time to accept that I had feelings for men. I spent most of my early twenties burying these feelings because I felt bad about them. I've got a boyfriend now and it feels normal and natural. I kind of regret all that wasted time, but it just took me longer than some others, I suppose, and I'm happy that I've come through all that and am now content with who I am.' John, 29

For hundreds of years, gay men have suffered oppression because of their sexuality. Thankfully, today we are in a much better position, where many gay men can enjoy an openly gay lifestyle that is accepted as a natural and normal part of the fabric of society. Being gay today certainly does not carry the stigma it used to.

However, that might be more the case in certain parts of the country and sections of society. Many gay men still experience difficulties, not only in coming to terms with their sexuality but also from the homophobia they experience through living a gay life. Many gay men still choose not to be open about their sexuality because of their fear of prejudice and hostility. So being gay today is certainly not easy for everyone.

Surveys show that most gay men realise that they are gay somewhere between the ages of 12 and 17.[1] But this realisation usually takes time – years, in some cases – to really hit home. What most gay guys first remember is somehow feeling different from other boys or not being interested in the same things as the other boys of their age. Often this feeling of 'just being different' can continue up to and through adolescence. This can lead to confused emotions about who you are, especially if you start to experience sexual feelings towards boys or men. It can be a scary and unpleasant time. Many feel isolated because no one else around them seems to be going through the same experiences. Many also suffer bullying, including name-calling and even physical abuse.

WHAT'S GAY ANYWAY?

'I don't call myself gay because I go with women too – always have. I don't have a partner right now but in the past I've had both girlfriends and boyfriends – and they know that I'm "bi". Sometimes I feel like being with a woman and sometimes a man. I can't say who I'll fall in love with.'
Jerome, 32

In the late 1940s, Alfred Kinsey, one of the most famous sex researchers, claimed that sexuality was not a simple matter of being straight or gay but could encompass a range of sexual feelings towards members of the same and the opposite sex. He found that while some men were 100 per cent straight and some were 100 per cent gay, there were many who were aroused by both men and women to varying degrees.

There are men who have relationships only with men and others who have relationships with both sexes. The results of studies vary regarding the exact numbers, but most show that up to 1 in 10 men (10 per cent) who have sex with other guys call themselves bisexual because they also have sex with women.[2]

People can love or hate labels. To some, they are important because they make them feel part of a group. Others find labels restricting, either because they don't like to be 'put into a box' or because they feel they are changing, and so a single label can't apply to them all the time. There are lots of labels to choose from. As well as 'gay', there is 'straight', 'bi', 'queer' and 'MSM' (men who have sex with men). Although some men prefer to be called 'gay', defining 'gay' is a personal thing. For some, it is about having sex with other guys. For others, it's about having sexual feelings towards them, or about living life as an 'out' gay man.

WHY AM I GAY?

When dealing with thoughts and feelings that they might be gay, many men want to know if they were *born* gay or *became* gay, for example, as a result of their upbringing. There is no simple answer to this question. Often the debate is geared around the questions 'Are you born gay?' or 'Do you become gay?': a 'natural' cause or a 'biological' cause through your upbringing (nurture).

There is research to show that it's your genetic makeup (the mixture of the genes you got from your mother and father) that plays a big role in determining your sexuality. For example, studies show that there is a 40–50 per cent chance that if one identical twin brother is gay the other will be too, and if you're gay then there is a higher chance that someone else in your family is, or was, gay. So for a while there has been the hunt for the 'gay gene'. Over the last few years the entire human genetic makeup has been scanned and research suggests that genetic patterns on three different chromosomes are shared amongst many gay men and that these may influence homosexuality. But a gay gene probably won't be found, because sexuality is likely to be controlled by several genetic regions acting together and not just one gene.

Apart from genetic factors biology is also likely to play a big role in sexuality. Although you can't always compare animals and humans there are lots of studies that show that homosexuality exists in other animals like birds, dolphins, sheep, bats...the list goes on. Some studies have found that a particular area of a sheep's brain that controls sexual behaviour is bigger in heterosexual sheep compared to homosexual sheep. And there is some early research that suggests there may be similar differences in human males – but the researchers say more work is needed to be sure. What causes these differences in size of parts of the brain is not really known. Some say it may be due to environmental influences such as hormone levels whilst a baby grows in the womb.

For some there are potential problems with scientists looking to prove that sexual orientation is down to biology or genetics. They worry that if a genetic cause is confirmed it may stigmatise being gay as a kind of illness and lead some to try to find a 'cure', perhaps through genetic screening. Others find the research into biology or genetics reassuring because it proves what they feel – that they were born gay and it is not a lifestyle choice.

However, although genetics and biology contribute an important role in sexuality, there is research on the other side of the debate that psychologists and psychiatrists have carried out into the role that upbringing plays in sexuality. There are lots of ideas regarding the influence that home environment and parental influence have on being gay. Commonly held views include the theory that having an overbearing mother or not having a father figure during childhood might cause you to grow up to be gay. Often these ideas do not bear close scrutiny. There are many straight guys who grew up with powerful mother figures and without dads. Until a few decades ago homosexuality was seen as a psychiatric disorder – called at one time 'sexual deviance'. There were even severe psychological treatments – some even had electric shock therapy – to try to cure men of their gayness.

Nowadays most would agree that sexuality is more likely to be down to a mix of your genetics, biological influences and upbringing – that is, both nature and nurture. Your sexuality is a complicated matter and so what makes it the way it is is likely to be equally complicated.

HOW MANY GAYS ARE THERE IN THE VILLAGE?

Calculating the exact numbers of gay men in the country is not as easy as it might seem. One thing is for sure, though, you are not alone! It's hard to know the exact numbers because being gay means different things to different people. The National Survey of Sexual Attitudes and Lifestyles in Britain[3] reported that, of those questioned:

* Nearly 1 in 12 men (8.4 per cent) had had a sexual experience with another man at some point in their lives.
* Nearly 1 in 16 men (6.3 per cent) had had sex (that is, genital contact) with another man at some point in their lives.
* Nearly 1 in 40 men (2.6 per cent) had had sex with another man in the last five years.

It's impossible to know whether there are more gay people around today than there were in the past. What's clear is that gay men and gay lifestyles are more 'out' and visible than ever before. There are more gay role models on the TV, and in films and magazines, and more gay men live openly gay lives in the public eye. There have also been lots of advances in gay rights, such as civil partnerships and laws prohibiting discrimination against gays that make it easier to live life as an 'out' gay man.

KEY POINTS
* Sexuality is probably not the black and white issue that some people think.
* What makes you gay is likely to be a mix of your genes and your upbringing.
* It's hard to be certain just how many men are gay, but a study found that nearly 3 in 100 men surveyed reported having had sex with another guy in the previous five years.

TWO

COMING OUT AND FINDING YOUR SCENE

'I think my parents knew all along that I was gay. I remember telling my mum quite casually one day when I was 17 that I had a boyfriend. She wasn't fazed at all – or didn't seem to be. I know that it can be really hard for some people to tell their parents, but it was quite natural for me. Saying that, I think my mum told my dad and he's never mentioned it!'
Simon, 19

Perhaps the biggest dilemma that gay guys face is whether to be open and honest about their sexuality because of the fear that they will face hostility, homophobia or that their friends and family will reject them. Many find the decision one of the biggest challenges they have to face, but once they make it, it is often a huge relief. For others, the announcement that they are gay is something that just happens and is not a major issue.

Whether or not you choose to come out – and if you do, when, how and who to tell – is a personal decision. Some guys come out just as soon as they realise they are gay, often when they are still young. For others, this decision takes years. Some never come out at all. Everyone has their own views on this. If you search the Internet for others' experiences of coming out you can read stories from men the world over – each one different from the next.

BUT WHY COME OUT?

Most gay men say it is a relief to tell others how they feel. For many, myself included, it can feel as if a massive weight has been lifted off the shoulders. There is a sense of relief that a secret has finally been let out and all the pretending to be someone you're not can stop. Battling with your sexuality can not only be emotionally exhausting but can also damage your confidence and sense of self worth. Most guys spend some time covering up or even lying about how they feel, trying to fit in and play the straight role. Some do so for years, and this can make relationships with friends and family strained.

For some men, denying who they are can make it much more difficult to have sexual relationships, not only because of the need to cover up but also through the guilt this causes. So, for most guys, coming out has a positive effect on how they feel about themselves and their relationships. It makes it possible for them to express and discover who they truly are. It gives them the possibility of finally living a full life where they are free to experience all human emotions.

THE STAGES

No one would say that coming out is easy, and there are risks involved. For some people, such as family and friends, the news can be so unwelcome that it may cause a strain – even a complete breakdown – in your relationship with them. You will choose who to come out to, and when. More men are out to friends only, and not to work colleagues or family members. That works for them. Who you choose to tell will depend on your own particular circumstances. If you need advice, there is lots of help out there, people to see or call, no matter what your

HOW 'OUT' ARE YOU?

A survey of more than 16,000 gay men across the UK[1] found that only about 3 in 10 (33 per cent) were 'out' to almost everyone – friends, work and family – while more than 1 in 9 (12 per cent) were completely 'in' to all these people.

Many minority communities place an especially strong emphasis on family tradition and marriage, making coming out particularly hard. Being gay can mean there will be no marriage and no children, and hence no continuation of the family line. This disruption of the family tree can be an important issue in all families but is especially so in minority communities. So coming out runs the risk of being excluded from that whole community. It is not surprising then that, compared to white guys, black and Asian men are less likely to be 'out' to their friends, work colleagues and family. In fact, only 1 in 5 gay black men (20 per cent) and 1 in 9 gay Asian men (11 per cent) say they are fully out, compared to over 1 in 3 white gay men (36 per cent). Conversely, 27 per cent of Asian gay men and 15 per cent of black gay men say they are completely 'in' compared to only 11 per cent of white gay men.[2]

situation. You may feel that no one is in the same boat as you but you will find that you are not alone.

Stage one: Coming out to yourself

'I think that the hardest step for me was that I could be okay with being gay. I remember thinking that unless I could be happy with who I was then there was no way that anyone else would be.' Adam, 27

Many gay men say that the first stage in their coming out was *coming out to themselves*. This stage involves accepting yourself and feeling good about who you are – and the fact that you are gay. For some guys this is not an issue and they come to terms with their sexuality from an early age. For others, accepting themselves as being gay can be hard and can take years to come to terms with. There are many reasons for this, but a common factor may be that family or society has taught you that being gay is wrong or dirty and so you may hide or deny your feelings. Many gay men spend time wishing that their feelings are a phase they are going through and that will pass in time.

Accepting and learning to like yourself can be challenging but, according to many gay men, this is a crucial first step. Not liking the fact that you are gay is a kind of self-directed homophobia and so is never going to help you to feel happy about yourself. There are many voluntary agencies, local and on-line groups and telephone help lines you can contact for support who will help you to understand your sexuality and develop a positive attitude to who you are. Being gay is only a part of you – it is not the whole story. It will help to remember that you have your own unique personality and personal qualities that are nothing to do with your sexuality.

Stage two: Coming out to someone else

'He told me by writing me a letter – I wish I still had it! I was shocked at first but then we spoke about it and it was like, okay, so you're gay, so what?! I love my brother and I think we can be more honest with each other now.' Helen, 25

The next stage of coming out is to *tell someone else about how you feel*. This is normally a feeling you have inside you and you just want to share your news with someone. However, you need to give this step some thought. Think about who you trust and feel comfortable with and whether he or she will be supportive. Ask yourself why you want to do it. If you want to take this step simply because you feel ready and you are proud of who you are, then – great! But if your intention is to shock or hurt someone it is best to take another look at your motives.

Many choose a friend or sibling to tell or even write them a letter. But it can be a good idea to test the water first. There is probably little point in simply blurting out the news to someone who you think might have a problem with your being gay. You have to face the possibility that who you tell may not react well to the news. You could lose a friend, or they might tell others before you have a chance to. So plan ahead and pick a time that's right. The news may come as a surprise to some people, especially if you have been leading a straight life before, whereas others may have known all along. Either way, they're likely to have lots of questions for you – so be prepared.

Stage three: Coming out further

'I remember it was a Saturday evening. This was a pretty strange time for me to be ringing up. I must have sounded really flat because she asked me what was wrong. "I've got something to tell you," I said, already crying into the phone. [My mum] was so worried and concerned, I could hear it in her voice. "I can't tell you, I can't tell you," I said. "What is it, Mark? Are you ill? Are you okay? Tell me – it doesn't matter." I don't know where the words came from – "I'm in love ... with another man." What had been building up for so many years – I was 26 when I told her – suddenly was over. The phone was silent. "I want to come home," I said. "Yes, come home then." She was quiet so I could tell she was upset, but she had still asked me to come home.' Mark, 34

Being openly gay – to your family and colleagues – isn't for everyone. Each gay man has his own unique challenges and so will decide for himself just how 'out' he wants to be.

Coming out to your family: Telling your family that you are gay can be the biggest hurdle of all. There are many gay men who lead gay lifestyles and have boyfriends – often for years and years – and yet are not out to their families. Because of all the covering up they have to do, they lead a double life that can be mentally and physically exhausting. For a start, there is the problem of avoiding questions regarding girlfriends and marriage. It's natural to worry about the disappointment your parents may feel, or that your mum and dad will be so upset they will never want to see you again. As previously mentioned, in many minority communities especially, with their strong emphasis on family tradition and marriage, coming out is particularly difficult. It carries the risk of being excluded from that whole community.

Some gay men start by telling a brother or sister and then gauge their reaction. How far you go is a personal choice and one you will make only when you are ready. If you decide to tell your family then aim to break the news to them in a compassionate way and be prepared for the questions that will follow. You may have a good idea of how your family will react but all families take the news differently.

Your family will need time to digest the knowledge that you are gay. Over time, many do learn to accept it. But how long this takes differs, and it is a fact that some never do. For many gay men, the knowledge that they are now being honest about their sexuality and the relief that comes from being able to stop pretending to be someone they are not, outweighs the pain and anguish that their announcement may cause.

Coming out at work: Many gay men prefer to keep their personal lives and work lives separate – just as many straight men do. So whether or not you choose to be 'out' at work is a personal decision and one you need to take some time to think about. Some gay men know, or fear, that they work in a homophobic environment or that coming out will prejudice their careers. You'll know instinctively what is best for you. But there are now laws against discrimination on grounds of sexuality that should protect you if you feel that you are facing harassment or unfair treatment at work because you are gay.

Coming out to your doctor: Most gay men see their GP as often as they need to but studies show that up to 1 in 2 (50 per cent) does not tell his GP that he is gay and 2 in 5 (40 per cent) do not want their GP to know.[3] Some gay men worry that they'll get a hostile reaction from their doctor and it's certainly true that some have had a negative or mixed reaction when they have been honest about their sexuality. Others worry about how the information will be recorded in their notes and, especially in smaller towns, are concerned that other members of staff in the surgery may find out and spread gossip.

In the past, doctors and other health professionals have been shown to be just as homophobic as many people in society as a whole. But as the attitude of society changes so the attitudes of most doctors are changing too. Studies show that most gay men who come out to their doctors are glad that they did so and did not get the homophobic reaction that they feared. Your sexuality could have an impact on your health. If you have a regular doctor then not being open about your sexuality could be bad for you. It can stop you from building a meaningful relationship with your doctor or focusing attention on health issues or concerns that are specific to you as a gay man.

PREJUDICE AND HOMOPHOBIA

The fear of homophobia stops many gay men living an openly gay life. Many guys say that they were bullied at school for being gay or being thought to be gay. It is still an unfortunate reality that gay men do suffer from discrimination. In one survey, around 1 in 3 guys (34 per cent) questioned said he was verbally abused in the preceding year by strangers, work colleagues, or family or friends, and 1 in 20 (5 per cent) on public transport.[4] And 1 in 14 (7 per cent) said he had actually been physically attacked because of his sexuality. The risk of this happening varies according to where you live – it seems to be more common in the north of England, for example. So it is not surprising that nearly 1 in 2 gay men (50 per cent) surveyed said he would not show affection to another man in public because of the fear of being insulted or harmed in some way.[5]

Gay men are reluctant to report this kind of hate crime. But it is important they do so. Apart from being a very unpleasant experience, the acceptance of prejudice and homophobia can affect how you feel about yourself and may even lead to anxiety or depression. It can certainly make you feel bad about who you are and about your sexuality. Most police forces are now encouraging gay victims of hate crimes to come forward and also provide support services for those who have been affected in this way.

The law has now advanced enough to offer the lesbian, gay and bisexual community full protection against discrimination. The Commission for Equality and Human Rights, set up in 2006, is a body that promotes and protects equality for all – across gender, race, sexuality or disability. It can protect you against discrimination in all areas of life – at school, at work and at home.

FINDING YOUR SCENE

'I started going out at 16 but now laugh at how I was to start with. I just had no idea and was so naïve. It took me weeks to pluck up the courage. I just went to a gay pub one weekday night and it was so terrible. I felt sure everyone was looking at me – but they probably weren't. And there was no one there like me at all – it was full of middle-aged guys drinking pints!'
Adrian, 17

When many men first start to have feelings that they might be gay their instinct is to look around for images or role models of what it means to be gay. Many guys of my generation were presented either with the image of a very effeminate guy mincing his way around, or one with a handle-bar moustache and hairy chest, straight out of the Village People. Today, you might think that the typical gay image is a well-dressed, gym-toned guy who is great at interior decorating and goes pubbing and clubbing every weekend.

But it's a myth that all gay men are the same. Take a close look and you'll see that gay men look and behave very differently and come in all shapes, sizes and colours. They have different jobs, personalities and interests. We're just as diverse as our straight counterparts.

Naturally, everyone likes to find friends who share their interests. So most gay men go on the pub, bar and club scene – at least for a while. The choice you have will depend on where you live. Most find out what's available in their area through the Internet, gay magazines or voluntary organisations and agencies for gay men. The gay scene is bigger in the major cities across the country but smaller towns too may have at least one gay pub. The first step into the gay world can be daunting as well as exciting, and most soon find others who they want to hang out with. You'll soon discover that the scene is as diverse as the gay community itself. So whether you're a 'club kid', 'biker boy', 'bear', 'leather daddy', 'drag queen' or 'circuit queen' you'll find people you like.

Some gay men prefer to be 'non-scene' and stay away from gay pubs and clubs, or they may have been on the scene but have become tired of pubbing and clubbing and can't wait to get off it! Mainstream gay culture can be harsh and bitchy, with too many guys so keen to fit in that they feel threatened by anyone who is different. So if you don't have the 'right' body or skin colour then you might feel that you're being left out. Some guys even get abuse from other gay guys about the way they look or how they act. It's strange that gay guys can be prejudiced towards other gay men. But it's often those who dish out the bitchy comments, and who seem to fit in so well, that feel the most insecure.

Some gay men find the scene too commercialised or shallow or just not to their taste. It's quite likely that if you've been going to the same pubs and clubs for a while you might want to explore different directions in your life. While the gay scene can give you support and confidence, after a while you may feel that you no longer need it to give you an identity and seek to find a little independence from it. If you are a guy who doesn't click with the scene or has just become tired of it, there are plenty of opportunities to do something different and to join groups to do it with. For example, there are websites that can help you (see Further Information, Resources, Websites and Organisations, page 263). Some feature massive directories of gay groups involved in sport, travel, cars – in fact loads that might interest you and help you meet other gay men with similar interests.

KEY POINTS

* Coming out can be daunting, but for most it's not as bad as they imagined.
* Most gay men say that coming out gives them a huge sense of relief that they can stop pretending to be someone they are not.
* Lots of organisations and websites offer advice and support on how to come out.
* You will decide how out you want to be: some men prefer to be out only to friends but stay in the closet at work or to their relatives.
* Gay men are as diverse as their straight counterparts and there are lots of different gay scenes to choose from where you can find friends.

THREE

CRUISING AND CASUAL SEX

'I just want to have casual sex right now. I'm looking for no-strings fun! I don't want a relationship – I'm too young – but if I met someone along the way I wouldn't say no!' Johnny, 24

Casual sex, one-night stands, anonymous sex – call it what you want – plays a part in many, but not all, gay men's lives. A survey in 2004 of gay men across England reported that about 1 in 5 (20 per cent) said he'd had one partner in the previous year, 1 in 4 (25 per cent) had had between two and four partners, 1 in 4 (25 per cent) had had between two and 12 partners, and 1 in 4 (25 per cent) had had more than 13 partners.[1] This was a big spread and so you can see that there is no 'normal' amount of sex that gay men have. Also it is important to bear in mind that this survey was filled in by gay men who were either at a gay pub, or a gay festival, or visiting a gay website – so these figures may be an overestimate and not representative of the gay community as a whole.

Casual sex might be what you want. For some it is sex for sex's sake. But for others casual sex can mean much more and will often lead on to more. It's pretty common for gay men to have sex on the first date – this can often lead to follow-up meetings and even lasting relationships. The term 'casual sex' can sound like something throwaway, but it can be intensely emotionally charged and intimate – so the word 'casual' often does not do it justice.

You may not feel ready for a full-on relationship, or you might want to have fun with different guys to find out what you're into and to build up your sexual confidence and ability. Casual sex plays a role in the sexual lives of most gay guys, and although I'm not saying you have to do it too, it can help you explore sexually.

While casual sex can be hugely satisfying on many fronts, don't expect it to always be good sex. There will be disappointments along the way. You can try to avoid these by finding out what your guy is into and see if that matches with you. Don't go with anyone who you're not sure you fancy. If you find that you're not into the sex you're having then it's best to be honest and just leave. Every man who has had casual sex knows that sometimes it works and other times it doesn't.

Some guys meet other guys for casual sex on a regular basis. They are called 'sex mates' or 'fuck buddies'. They know that they are meeting for sex alone and that a relationship is not on the cards. This kind of set-up can work well if you're both honest and open about what you want – and stick to the plan.

CRUISING

Gay men look for or cruise for sex virtually everywhere, from the street to cyber space. In a 2004 survey, over 2,000 London gay men, most aged between 20 and 40, were asked where they had met their most recent partner.[2] This is what they reported:

Meeting site	Percentage of gay men
Bar or club	43.0
Internet website	16.0
Sauna	9.8
Back room or sex club	6.1
Party/social group	5.4
Cruising ground/cottage	3.5
University/college/work	3.4

Gym	2.3
Dating agency	0.8
Telephone chat line	0.6
Other	9.1

Where you meet your partners can have implications for your heath and safety.

Bars and clubs

Bars and clubs are the most common places where gay men meet. Depending on where you live, there can be bars for 'club kids', for 'trendies', for the 'muscle boy crowd', for older guys, larger guys and your standard gay pub that's for everyone. If you are new to the scene then entering a bar can seem intimidating. But remember that everyone else is there to be sociable too.

A drink can help you to relax and give your confidence a boost. But too much and you're likely to lose your edge and are more likely to have unsafe sex and so pick up and pass on a sexually transmitted infection (STI), including HIV.

For most gay men, cruising in a bar or club comes by instinct. But about 1 in 5 (20 per cent) gay men says that he needs help with how to do it.[3] Many gay men find it hard to make the first move or don't know how to respond when someone shows an interest in them. Here is a step-by-step guide that may help:

1 Simply positioning yourself near to the guy you like is the first step and can be a sign that you're interested in him.
2 The next step is to look at him. Don't just catch his eye and turn away – that shows no interest. Take a longer look and, if you can manage it, give him a smile before you turn away. Hold your smile for a moment or two after you turn away – this shows that you are friendly and approachable.
3 If he's interested in you he should return your look.
4 If you got a smile back from yours the hard work is over. It's now up to you – or him – to open the conversation. Don't try too hard at this stage. General conversational openers are usually the best, and if you click with the guy then some connection or shared interest will usually come up.

Internet

It's not surprising that the Internet is number two in the list of meeting places. Many gay men are members of one of the popular gay Internet sites, and most use it to find sexual partners. A survey of 15,000 gay men across England in 2005 showed that 60 per cent had an Internet profile.[4] The Internet allows you to view hundreds of profiles or search for your particular type in your city, county or across the world from the comfort of your own home. No wonder it is so popular!

There are many to choose from, but Gaydar.co.uk and Gay.com are the most popular. Logging on and creating a profile is very easy – and you can pay or not, according to the level of service that you'd like. But take care when using the Internet: you can get addicted to it. A study of men using gay Internet sites found that 3 per cent of respondents were addicted to doing so, although this is unlikely to be representational of all gay men in the UK.[5]

Be cautious, too, about believing what you see and read. Many guys say that other guys show false pictures, or pictures don't match the reality, or some write complete fiction about themselves, such as knocking years off their ages or pretending to be someone they are not.

If you do hook up with someone it is a good idea to choose a public place for your first meeting so that you can check each other out and see if your 'profiles' match. It's also a good idea to let someone know where you are going or perhaps get them to ring you to check that everything is okay.

Saunas, back rooms and sex clubs

Saunas, back rooms and sex clubs are places that guys go specifically to have sex. How many there are in your area will depend on where you live, but generally they are more common in larger cities.

Check the back pages of any gay magazine and you'll find a listing of saunas. Most work the same way: you go in, pay your money, get a locker to keep your clothes in and are given a towel. You'll soon get the hang of what goes on by just having a walk around. There are generally a number of saunas, steam rooms, often a video lounge or a network of cubicles where guys go for sex. But there is some sauna etiquette. It's all about picking up on cues of interest. You'll find your partner or partners by checking them out or simply making a move on them. If a guy is eyeing you up or makes a move on you and you're not interested then don't return his looks, or just get up and move away. The same goes if there are more than two guys playing together. If you try to join in you'll soon get the message if they are interested or not.

Back rooms are more common in Europe, but there are a few in the UK. They are darkened rooms or corridors that you wander through or more often feel your way around! You need a good sense of touch because you really don't know what you're going to come up against. Some guys hang around outside to see who's going in.

Sex clubs are like back rooms, but may be more specialised – catering for, say, uniform guys, or they may have other dress codes such as Y-fronts or boots only. Most have changing facilities. Again, the listings in most gay publications will give you an idea of what kind of club it is. There will often be a porn room and cubicles that you can go to for sex.

It's possible that in one of these places you'll have sex with more than one man. The more men you have sex with, the greater the risk that you will pick up an STI. You're likely to be there because you're feeling horny, or you might still be high from a night out, or you might have been drinking. All these factors make it more likely that you will have risky sex.

Condoms and lubricating gel (lube) are likely to be available free at these places, but it is always advisable to take your own supply. In a sauna, it is a good idea to tuck some condoms under your locker key wristband.

Cruising grounds/cottages

Cruising grounds and 'cottages' are public places where guys go to meet other guys to have sex with. In the past, public toilets were the most common places but now it's more likely to be a public park. Part of the buzz that guys get from having this kind of sex is the sense of danger and the fact that they might be found out. Cruising is usually done at night and so this adds to the sense of excitement and the unexpected.

But cruising grounds and cottages are not without serious risk. Many gay men are robbed, so it's wise not to take valuables, or to keep your wallet in a zipped pocket. Or better still, leave it at home.

You might have had a few drinks before going to give you a bit of confidence, or may even be high on drugs. But these can lead you to taking risks with your health that you might not otherwise take. On a practical level, many such areas are poorly lit and so following safe sexual practices can be even more of a challenge.

TIPS FOR SAFER CRUISING

If you fancy cruising a public park, think about the potential dangers. You could be attacked and/or robbed and run the risk of life-threatening injuries, permanent disability or worse. That said, if you still decide you want to go ahead there are a few dos and don'ts to bear in mind that might help to minimise the risks:

* Most guys go cruising alone, but you could try persuading a friend to go with you or at least tell someone where you are going.

* Don't wear expensive jewellery or watches. A mugger might mark you down as an easy victim and follow you into the park.

* Don't carry credit cards or large amounts of cash, and never 'flash your cash' – again, you might be targeted by muggers.

In the eyes of the law, homosexual sex is *only* legal if it involves no more than two consenting adults (both aged 16 or over) and takes place in private. Whether or not a public park will be regarded as 'private' will depend on a variety of factors such as the time of day, the level of lighting, and the likelihood that another person may arrive on the scene. In other words, an out-of-the-way area of a little-used park after midnight *may* be regarded as private. Hyde Park at noon on August Bank Holiday Monday most certainly will not!

However, the law is clear as far as public toilets are concerned, and if you are caught having sex in one you will almost certainly end up at the police station. Bear in mind, too, that sex with someone under 16 is illegal, regardless of consent. In a dimly lit park or toilet it might be difficult to tell the person's age but the onus will be on you to prove you had good reason to believe he was older.

WHEN CRUISING GETS OUT OF CONTROL

Quick, anonymous sex can be a part of a healthy sex life but it can stop you forming deeper, more emotional relationships, and can get out of control. Cruising for sex can even become an addiction. However, there are ways that you can learn to modify your behaviour and so if you feel that your cruising is becoming a problem it is best to seek help (see page 223).

Chat lines

Relatively few guys hook up after being on a chat line. Listings in the back of most gay magazines give a long list of numbers to choose from.

With no physical contact there is no risk to your health but there could be a risk to your bank balance. Check the rates – you may find that that hour has cost you far more than it was worth.

Other meeting places

About 1 in 10 guys (10 per cent) meets a partner in none of the places mentioned above. We all know that gay men cruise and meet everywhere – the café, the street, the beach and the supermarket, to name a few.

DOS AND DON'TS OF PICKING UP CASUAL PARTNERS

* Do choose a public place to meet, such as a pub, if meeting someone for the first time.

* Do make sure someone knows where you are.

* Do have your mobile with you at all times and some cash on you so you can get home.

* Do make sure you always carry condoms, regardless of whether you plan to have sex or not.

* Don't accept a drink from a stranger unless you see it being poured at the bar. Drinks can be spiked with drugs that you can't taste, which can make you drowsy, and there are cases of guys who have been raped as a consequence.

* Don't leave drinks unattended, or don't drink them if you have because you risk them getting spiked.

* If you decide to go back to his place or are inviting him to yours, try and let a friend know you are going. It's hard to know for sure if you can trust someone but trust your instincts and don't base your decisions on how horny you feel!

* Drinking and drugs can cloud your judgement and so can add to the risk of picking someone up for casual sex.

* Don't take unnecessary risks with someone you've just met – like agreeing to bondage or risky sex games. For these a good level of trust in needed – something that is hard to have if you've only just met.

PAYING FOR SEX

'I have a good job and have a great lifestyle. Yeah, I am looking for a boyfriend still, but until that happens, I want to have good sex – and with a hot guy. The easiest way for me to get it, when I want it, is to pay for it.'
Edward, 35

Some surveys show that 1 in 20 gay men (5 per cent) pays for sex.[6] Most often, escorts are found through the Internet but many are also listed in the back pages of many gay magazines. Whatever your attitude towards prostitution, if you are going to use escorts then be aware of the risk this poses to your health.

It is fairly simple to organise a meeting as most escorts have a web address or mobile telephone number for you to contact. Most are willing to come to your place or for you to visit them. When you do make contact, be sure to ask that he provides what you are looking for and confirm the price. You'll be paying for his time – usually by the hour, but overnights are possible – and rates will vary according to whether you go to his place or he comes to yours. If you're looking for anything more than oral or anal sex – such as fetish or other types of sex – it is likely to cost you more. If you want your escort to ejaculate, that costs extra too. Longer sessions and even days or trips are possible – but again at a price. Be wary that the pictures you see may not be the reality you get on your doorstep. Just like Internet dating, there are guys who use false pictures downloaded from the Internet, so if you don't like what you see – don't let him in!

It might seem obvious, but when an escort calls round you are not going to be his only client. Most will insist on using condoms for anal sex. But not all escorts will insist on condoms for oral sex – and you can still pick up many STIs from sucking his penis without protection.

Paying for sex is not illegal as long as the escort is at least 18 years of age.

KEY POINTS

* Most men find partners by going to bars or clubs, but the next most popular way is through the Internet.

* When using the Internet for dating, be aware that some men use fake profiles and so won't match up to what you are expecting.

* Saunas, back rooms, sex clubs or cruising grounds are places where men go specifically for casual sex.

* These places can put you at high risk of STIs.

* Wear condoms for sex. And always take your own with you.

* Cruising grounds can be a target for muggers and thugs, so take precautions.

* Paying for sex is not illegal so long as your escort is at least 18.

FOUR

RELATIONSHIPS

'I've always wanted a boyfriend – for as long as I can remember. I know many of my friends don't but I suppose seeing my parents so happy together makes me want something similar. I've had lots of fun being single but I'm ready to settle down now and want to build a life with some-one – someone who I'll spend the rest of my life with and someone I can get old and fat with!' Suki, 30

Gay men can have a reputation for spending their lives cruising for sex, being single and having lots of casual partners. But surveys show that about 1 in 2 gay guys (50 per cent) has a regular partner.[1] When these guys were asked how long they had been together, the average length of time reported was about three years.

There are lots of reasons why guys decide to form relationships. Some guys tire of the casual scene and want something deeper and longer term. Relationships can also provide stability and support. But for most, it comes down to a simple matter of enjoying sharing your life with someone else and being loved and loving someone else.

Gay men don't necessarily run their sexual and emotional lives along the same lines as straight guys. We tend to be more flexible and open – and perhaps more realistic about relationships and their possibilities. There is also a greater variety of gay relationships – such as open relationships, relationships with more than one guy, and so on. Finding the relationship type that suits you is important and you shouldn't feel that you need to fit any particular model.

When you think about gay couples, what image comes to mind? You might think of two men who have modelled themselves on the traditional straight couple: one more masculine, the other more feminine. Maybe you imagine a couple who are like clones, similar in personality and appearance. But, in reality, you can't really predict who will go with whom. You may think you prefer a particular type of man, but who really attracts you may, in the end, be very wide of the mark. Furthermore, you might have your eye on a particular kind of man, but you can't be sure what type *he* goes for. His type may be a long way from what you might imagine. Many gay couples are made up of guys from different racial, cultural and social backgrounds. Age differences are common too. Many gay couples celebrate these differences and they can even be a predictor of success in a relationship.

Finding 'Mr Right' can be a challenge – in fact about 1 in 4 gay men (25 per cent) wants help with finding a boyfriend.[2] There is no easy answer to this problem; often experience and practice are the only solutions.

It is likely that, if you're finding it hard to find or maintain a relationship, the issue might lie at your door rather than being the fault of every guy you meet. Some men don't find 'Mr Right' because as soon as they start a relationship all they can see are the faults in their partner. For one reason or another, the partner is never quite good enough. Having a relationship is all about taking the risk of being open to another person. Gay men often shy away from this because they have spent years covering up how they feel and fear being hurt or rejected. Many find it easier to avoid the depth of emotion and intimacy needed for a relationship and prefer the buzz of casual or short-term relationships. So, the first step towards finding a relationship is to look inside yourself and decide whether you are ready for one and whether or not it's what you really want.

There is no ideal model of what a gay relationship looks like. But having some understanding of how a relationship might work out over the years is important. Knowing what to expect might help you over any sticky patches.

THE DEVELOPMENT OF A RELATIONSHIP

A 1996 study revealed that gay relationships develop in stages.[3] Although these stages are not set in stone, the researchers found that the following sequence was a common experience for many gay couples:

* First year – blending. The relationship is full of excitement and full of sex!
* Two to three years – nesting. You start to become a true couple – perhaps even moving in together. Sexual activity may decline and you might start to see that your guy is not quite so perfect after all. Many guys get bored at this point and are tempted to move on and return to the exciting days of starting a new relationship.
* Four to five years – maintaining. If a gay couple has got this far they are probably starting to get the relationship balance right by being a couple but also maintaining their individuality. They start to build a sense of permanence into their relationship. The down side, however, is that this can be a time of sexual boredom. There can be the desire to show a little sexual independence.
* Five to ten years – building. Once they get over the hurdles encountered in the 'maintaining' stage of the relationship, gay couples get on with the job of sharing projects and longer-term aims in life, while still keeping their own lives 'alight'. They become more tolerant of their partner and show plenty of respect for each other.
* Ten to twenty years – establishing. Each partner now loosens his grip and is less possessive of the other. While in general this is a good thing, partners can begin to take each other for granted.
* Over twenty years – renewing. Medal time for sure! The risk that the relationship will fall apart is now very low. Couples reflect on all the things they did together bringing a renewed sense of meaning to the relationship.

Many gay couples say the two most important threads running through a relationship are good communication and independence, and often the only way to solve problems in a relationship is to discuss how you're feeling and talk through any difficulties between you. If you bottle up your emotions your partner may not realise that things aren't going right.

While having a boyfriend is important for many guys, as soon as some find a partner they can start to lose themselves in that relationship. In the short-term, that is natural and expected – falling in love is all-consuming. But, in relationship terms, two halves don't make a whole and forgetting who you are, and losing touch with friends and family, can put a lot of pressure on a gay relationship. So it's important to keep a degree of independence by retaining a strong sense of who you are as an individual.

The law is now on the side of gay couples. Since December 2005 same-sex couples can form a legally recognised civil union that gives them the same rights as straight couples over issues such as inheritance, tax and visiting rights in hospital. More information can be found in Further Information, Resources, Websites and Organisations (see page 263).

SEX AND YOUR RELATIONSHIPS

Sex plays a central role in any relationship and is likely to be what brought you both together in the first place. Especially with gay relationships, when most gay guys have other guys as friends, what makes the essential difference between a good friend and a lover or partner is sex.

In the first year, you will probably have a full sex life and are likely to feel excited and crazy with passion. But for most gay couples the pace and excitement you felt for each other in the early stages naturally declines over time. That doesn't mean the sex is not so good any more. It can get better. Many find that what replaces the lust of the early years is greater trust and a deepening of the meaning of sex as a way to communicate. So this new emotional aspect to sex compensates for any lessening of passion. Couples who have been together for a while are also more likely to experiment, trying out new things to add spice and adventure to their sex lives.

If you are not willing to put effort into maintaining a varied sex life then you risk boredom setting in. A declining sex life can just be about sex alone but can also be a sign of a deeper problem with the relationship. As your relationship develops your sex life needs to change as well.

Some couples choose to keep their sex lives varied by having an 'open relationship', but if you are planning to have sex with someone other than your partner it is best to be honest from the start; certainly better that way than waiting until one of you brings home a sexually transmitted infection.

Successful open relationships don't just happen by themselves, however, they require discussion and agreement. Without this, the core relationship is likely to fail. If you want to protect your emotional ties and your commitment to each other, you will need to decide exactly how you will manage sexual relationships outside your relationship. It is important to work out the ground rules together. It's quite common for one partner to be more in favour of an open relationship than the other. One partner might not understand why the other feels the need to go elsewhere for sex when he is quite happy with the way things are. Conflicts like this are difficult and can only be resolved through communication. Ground rules will only work if you are both prepared to stick to them. Jealousy and distrust can seriously damage the best relationships.

Many couples also bring in a third guy now and then to liven up their sex lives. This works for many but can bring up issues of jealousy and guilt. If you are planning on this, discuss what you both want from it, what you are hoping to do, what you will allow each other to do. This level of planning may seem to be going overboard and risks losing some of the spontaneity of sex, but you need to think these issues through clearly if you want to safeguard your relationship.

RULES SET BY COUPLES WHO 'PLAY OUTSIDE'

'We only play together – not alone.'

'We only play when we're abroad or on holiday.'

'I play around but, if he doesn't ask, I don't tell.'

'He can do what he wants as long as he doesn't get fucked – his arse is for me!'

'I can see a guy once – but only once. No follow-ups or second times are allowed!'

HIV AND RELATIONSHIPS

Some guys with HIV feel that there is little possibility of having a fulfilling and loving relationship, but this is not true. Any relationship is complicated, and adding in the fact that one of you is HIV positive means extra pressures – but these can be overcome. With the current rates of HIV in gay men, 'serodiscordant' relationships – where one guy has HIV and the other doesn't – are not uncommon. Recent studies of gay men across England show that about 1 in 20 (5 per cent) are in a serodiscordant relationship. Other studies show that these last as long as those between guys of the same HIV status.[4] It is clear then that many HIV positive men do form relationships and have happy, fulfilling emotional and sexual lives, where HIV is just part of the relationship – not the whole.

One problem that many men face is in deciding when to tell their partner. This is a difficult conversation to have at any time, as it can be tricky to gauge what the partner's reaction will be. When to break the news is a personal choice: at the start of a relationship, or after things have progressed a little. But some would argue that there is a moral duty to inform a partner of your HIV status if there is any possibility of sex that puts your partner at risk of picking up the virus – like anal or oral sex without a condom. Using a condom can reduce the risk of transmission but it can't eliminate the risk altogether. They can split or break. In addition, if you are HIV positive and don't inform a sexual partner of the fact, you risk prosecution if that person subsequently becomes infected (see page 87).

Many gay men with HIV fear or have experienced rejection and the loss of someone they care about after telling them about being positive. But there is no single way that men react to the news. Some find the issue too difficult to contemplate or simply don't want to deal with it and walk away. Others take it in their stride. There are issues that will need to be discussed, such as how the illness will affect a relationship. Although many men are living long and healthy lives as a result of antiretroviral drugs, they are living with a life-threatening illness and both partners will feel the burden of this. Perhaps one of the most challenging issues can be about sex and the worry that one of you having HIV will affect how much you enjoy sex and the kind of sex you want. When it comes to negotiating safer sex between two guys where one is HIV positive and the other is not, the best advice is to be well informed about the risks. Knowledge is your best protection. Anal sex poses the greatest risk of HIV transmission, but it can also be transmitted to the partner who is HIV negative if he performs oral sex on his partner with HIV, especially if he gets pre-cum or cum in his mouth (see page 180). Using condoms for anal and oral sex is therefore best.

Even if you know how to reduce the risk of passing on HIV through sex, it can be difficult to stick to the rules at all times. Some couples choose to stop using condoms because they believe this will make them closer, or may even think that it would be somehow easier if both were HIV positive anyway. These are difficult issues that can only be sorted out through honest and open discussion.

If both partners have HIV you might think there is no need to continue to follow safer sex practices. But there is research to show that you can become re-infected with your partner's strain of the virus – one that might be resistant to the medication you are taking and so attack your immune system.

It's important to remember that if, for some reason, you have sex that puts one of you at risk of transmitting HIV, there are medications available that may help to reduce the chances of contracting the virus (see page 177).

There is a lot of help and advice available for guys with HIV regarding relationships and other issues. Being able to discuss the fears and concerns that you both have will help you to work through problems as they arise. See Further

Information, Resources, Websites and Organisations (page 263) for websites offering advice and support for gay men affected by such issues.

KEY POINTS

* The type of partner you end up with may not be the one you were originally looking for, so be open to this possibility.
* There is no single model for a gay relationship. For some gay couples, the ideal is monogamy, but for others this is not the case.
* Relationships are not easy to maintain – they require working at. All relationships go through good times and not so good times.
* Communication is the key to keeping the relationship strong.
* Expect the sex within your relationship to change over time. Be prepared to make an effort if you want sex to stay fresh.
* When choosing open relationships, couples need to set clear ground rules to safeguard their health and relationship.
* If one partner has HIV it can create an additional challenge, but advice and support over all the issues involved can often provide the solution to any problems.

PART II

BODY
BEAUTIFUL

Ask yourself this question. Who do you think gets more pleasure out of sex – the gym god with hard abs and a tight butt or the average-looking guy who knows how his body works and how it can give him pleasure?

I hope you said the average-looking one! Yes, you might want to have sex with the good-looking man with the great body but it's actually those who know about their body who have the most sexual fun. It's common sense that the more you understand about your body the more confident you will feel about sex. Putting it another way, the less you know about your body, the less chance there is of you experiencing sexual pleasure. So the first and most basic step towards better sex is to know and understand your body – especially the parts you use most for sex. Not a bad reason to learn a bit of anatomy!

Another reason is that although when things are going right with our body we don't give it much thought, when things go wrong it can be very frightening – especially when it's anything to do with the parts we use for sex. By knowing more about yourself you will be able to spot when things aren't quite right and know what to do about it.

'I'm getting more and more worried about how I look. I started working out three years ago. I know that I look okay but the better I look the more and more I notice things that I don't like! I know they are small things that no one notices but I can't stop looking. In the gym I'm always checking out my abs and find it hard to pass a car now without looking at myself. To be honest, it's getting me down'. Jack, 22

When it comes to the body, gay men often come up against major hurdles. The biggest is that many are not satisfied with how they look. Although gay guys come in all shapes and sizes many don't judge their bodies against the average but against unrealistic images of other men, such as porn stars and guys who go to great lengths to build themselves up. It follows then that many gay men have high levels of dissatisfaction and anxiety regarding their bodies.

Why does this happen? Gay men have always been conscious of their appearance. This is not only a good way to attract attention – and potential part-ners – but also a way to build confidence that is often lacking through feelings of low self-esteem. There's also a lot of pressure on the gay scene to look a certain way, and naturally most guys just want to try to fit in.

Over the last fifteen years, the ideal body shape has changed to 'the beefier the better' and many gay men now go to great lengths to achieve their fantasy, including taking body-building drugs. Films and magazines promote this idealised image of what a gay body should be like.

However, deep down, every guy knows that although it's important to look good and to take care of your appearance, *looking good* does not automatically mean that you *feel good*. It might sometimes be hard to believe, but the guy who has a perfect body will have just as many hang-ups about it, or possibly more, than the guy with a more average body.

Feeling good about yourself will improve your self-confidence and so aiming to look the best you can is an important aim. But this can get to the stage where some men start to worry about their bodies when they don't need to. They may think they are overweight when they're not, or worry that they are not muscular enough when they are bulging already. In a few cases, this can become an unhealthy obsession that goes way beyond just being a little vain. Some men reach the stage where they are never satisfied with their body shape and never feel good about themselves. This is known as having a distorted body image.

Men who have this problem may think that some part of their body is too big or too small, when to other people they look normal or even great. It can be the nose, chin or the size of their chest, butt or penis. It fact, they may be dissatisfied with any part of their body and the slightest imperfection. They spend several hours of every day just thinking about it, and get into the habit of checking their appearance constantly. They spend a lot of time working on their appearance or toning their body and will often go to extremes to attain their idea of perfection. This can lead to them taking anabolic steroids (see page 239) to beef them up, or having cosmetic surgery. The sad thing is that no matter what they do they will never be fully satisfied with their appearance.

Developing a more positive self-image helps. That means developing a positive attitude towards yourself, valuing yourself and your abilities and not focusing on the negatives. This enhanced self-esteem comes from feeling in control of your life and making decisions in your life that you feel right about. In some cases, guys who are having difficulty with the way they see their body may need professional help, such as psychological counselling or antidepressant medication.

Such serious problems with body image are rare, but many guys probably place too much emphasis on how they look. So it's important to appreciate your body for what it is. One way is to learn how it works and how it can give you pleasure. This can help you focus on what you have – rather than what you haven't.

FIVE

SKIN, NIPPLES AND BEYOND

SKIN

Your skin covers the whole surface of your body, and has a central role in protecting you from injury and infection. It contains nerve endings that sense touch, temperature, pressure and pain – all sensations that are important to a sexual life.

The skin is comprised of three layers. The outer layer, the epidermis, is mostly made up of dead skin cells. New skin cells are made at the base of the epidermis and over about two weeks slowly mature, filling with a tough protein called keratin, flattening out, and dying as they rise to the surface. Once there, these skin cells flake off, for example, through contact with your clothes, and are replaced. About 5 per cent of the epidermis is made of cells containing melanin, the pigment that darkens the skin's colour. The more melanin you have, the darker your skin. In white people especially, these cells produce extra melanin when you sunbathe to give the skin a summer glow.

The middle layer, the dermis, contains nerve endings, blood vessels, oil glands and sweat glands. It also contains fibres of tough and flexible proteins called collagen and elastin. When your skin is touched, the nerve endings send messages to your brain. They are super sensitive and can tell the difference between the whole range of sensations from sharp to soft, hot to cold. The inner, subcutaneous, layer is mostly made up of fat for energy storage and to help keep the body warm.

When it comes to intimacy and sex, we use all of our senses – including sight, sound, smell and taste (see page 90), but for most people the sense of touch is the most important. For many men, touch – and feeling close to someone – is more important than sex itself.

Every man is wired up differently and has different pleasure points. For some, the lips are more sensitive and so for them kissing is particularly important. For others, the most sensitive areas are the testicles, or the anus, or the narrow strip of skin called the perineum, located between the testicles and the anus. For other guys, it's the nipples that crave more attention. Discovering your own and your partner's most sensitive areas will help you to focus on these pleasure-giving hot spots.

NIPPLES

Evolution has left men with nipples that don't serve an essential biological function as they do in women, in enabling them to breastfeed. But nipples do have an important function for men. They are sensitive and so can play a role in sexual arousal. For many men, nipple play is a key part of sex.

The nipple itself is surrounded by an area of sensitive skin called the areola. Most people have two nipples but some have what is called a third or accessory nipple.

Both the nipple and the areola can be considered erogenous organs because they are sensitive to touch and when stimulated the nipple becomes firm and erect. This also happens when your nipples get cold.

BIG BREASTS?

'I've met a guy who is really hot. He has a great body – really ripped – but he has got tits as well. They're not huge, but you can tell they are a bit swollen compared to the rest of him. It doesn't bother me, but I wonder if there is something wrong and whether I should mention it?' Tony, 32

In males, the condition of having abnormally enlarged breasts is called gynaecomastia. It is more common in adolescent boys or older men. The breast tissue enlarges, often in response to increased levels of the female hormone oestrogen (which all males have in small amounts) or a drop in the male hormone testosterone. In adult guys, the condition may be something they've had since puberty (physiological gynaecomastia), or may be due to other factors, such as the medications they are taking, or liver, kidney or testicular problems. It some men it is simply down to genetics. Often the condition doesn't need treatment unless it causes discomfort or embarrassment. The type of treatment given will depend on the underlying cause. Tablets may reduce the level of oestrogen in the body, or another option is surgery to remove excess breast tissue. If there is a discrete lump, this can be taken out via a small cut made around the nipple, or excess fatty tissue can be removed by liposuction. These operations leave small scars which fade in time. In the gay world, gynaecomastia is also known as 'bitch tits' and can be a side-effect of steroid drug use (see page 240).

In HIV-positive men, especially those on medication, gynaecomastia can be due to lipodystrophy. This is a condition in which fat deposits become re-located in the body. Sufferers can lose fat from some parts of the body, such as the cheeks and limbs, and gain it in other places, such as the chest, abdomen or back – in some cases, leading to severe disfigurement. This can be very distressing as guys become very self-conscious of how their looks have changed.

If a discrete lump can be felt in the breast, the possibility of breast cancer must be considered. Although rare, it does happen to men – 1 per cent of all breast cancers occur in males – so if you think that you are developing breasts, or feel any lumps in your chest, it's always really important to get them checked by a doctor.

PIERCING AND TATTOOS

'I had a tattoo done seven years ago, but I wasn't very happy with the result. It was a Celtic cross on my arm and was a bit of a botch job. I've never really liked the thing. It's all one colour (black), and about three inches by three inches. I found out about removal but it's really expensive, so I am going to try to have it made into a design that I like.' Matthew, 28

Body piercing and tattoos are popular ways of decorating the body. Piercing is also a way to increase sexual pleasure. Both methods have a history that goes back hundreds of years. Egyptian mummies have been found with tattoos on them, and Roman soldiers are said to have had nipple rings to hold their capes in place! Queen Victoria's son, Prince Albert, is claimed to have had a ring through his penis and hence his name was given to that particular form of piercing. (It is not named after her husband, also called Prince Albert, as is often supposed.)

Gay men often have piercings or tattoos for fashion, or because they just think it looks good. There's often a deeper reason, too, as a way to mark something significant in their lives or as a way to suggest that they've made a claim on their own bodies – a kind of statement of ownership. It also helps to be identified as part of a group. Guys are also very interested in heightening sensation during sex, and having a part of the body pierced is a popular way to enhance sexual pleasure.

A 2002 survey of more than 16,000 guys showed that just over 1 in 3 guys (33 per cent) had had some part of his body pierced, 1 in 4 piercings (25 per cent) was in the ear, and the next most common, around 1 in 10 (just over 10 per cent) was in the nipple. Face piercing was more common in younger guys, middle-aged guys preferred to have their nipples pierced and older guys were more likely to have genital piercing.[1]

Whatever your motivation, be sure to think it through and discuss it with others. Choose your body piercing artist/tattooist carefully: always go to someone reputable who is licensed to perform the procedure so that you know they will be vigilant about your health. Bear in mind that anaesthetic may not be available, so if you can't handle pain then a piercing or tattoo might not be for you. For some, the pain of the procedure is part of the ritual.

You can have almost any part of your body pierced. Commonly it's one or more of the following – ear, eyebrow, nose, lips, tongue, nipple, belly button, glans/foreskin, scrotum or perineum. Here is a list of the most popular:

Body part	Popularity (%)
Head/ears	26.2
Torso/nipples	11.3
Eyebrow	5.0
Scrotum/glans/foreskin/perineum	5.0
Navel	4.0
Tongue	3.6
Nose	2.4
Lips	1.3

Let's take a closer look at a couple of sites:

Nipples

Men often have their nipples pierced because they already enjoy a lot of sensation there or to increase the sensation they feel. It's one of the more painful places to have done. You usually start by having a thin rod or bar inserted into the piercing. If you want to play with the bar during sex, you'll need to wait until the piercing has healed and then have the original bar replaced with a thicker one or a ring.

Penis

There are lots of different types of penile piercing. The most famous – a Prince Albert (PA) – is a piercing of the glans, or head of the penis. This goes in through your urethra (the tube that carries urine out of the body) and out through the underside of the penis. Having a PA means that you could spray when you urinate – so the guy standing next to you at the urinals might not be too happy. The hole can close up if you remove the ring before the piercing has completely healed.

There are other types of penile piercing. In an ampalling, the bar runs from one side of your glans to the other. In an apadravya, the bar runs through your glans from top to bottom.

The heath risks of piercing

The following are some of the risks associated with body piercing:

* Infection. After piercing, keep the area clean, using an antibacterial soap or cleanser twice a day. If the piercing looks infected, leave the jewellery in place because this helps the piercing to drain. See your GP for some antibiotics.

* Bleeding. This doesn't happen often but if it does apply gentle pressure to the area. If the bleeding still doesn't stop you'll need to see a doctor.

* Allergy. Some guys are allergic to the piercing jewellery – especially if the item contains nickel – and may develop a rash around the piercing site. If this happens remove the item. You are likely to be okay with silver or gold jewellery.

* Sexually transmitted infections (STIs). Until the hole heals, which can take months, a piercing can be a route for picking up and passing on blood-borne infections such as hepatitis B and C and HIV.

* Surgery. All jewellery must be removed before any surgical operation can go ahead. This is because surgeons use an electric current to stop bleeding points and so there is a risk that your piercing jewellery may conduct the current, causing burning of the skin around the piercing site.

* Torn condom. Piercing jewellery should not normally tear a condom but, to be on the safe side, lay the jewellery to one side as you put the condom on.

* Scarring and closure. Piercing jewellery can generally be removed easily. If they are taken out early on then they may not leave a scar. The longer you have them in place, the more likely that a scar will form. Even if a piece of jewellery has been in place for years, if you don't wear it for a while the hole may close up and you'll need to have a fresh piercing made at the site.

Tattoos are made by injecting ink into the lowest layer of the skin, the dermis. It is done with a hand-held electric-powered device that works rather like a sewing machine. This is held a few centimetres away from the skin while one or more tiny needles move rapidly up and down, puncturing the skin and depositing the ink.

You can choose any design you like; you are limited only by the expertise of the tattoo artist or by your pain threshold! You should regard a tattoo as permanent as it is expensive to have one removed, so before you go ahead you need to be certain that you want to live with it!

The heath risks of tattoos

The following are some of the risks associated with tattoos:

* Infection. To produce a tattoo, the skin surface must be punctured hundreds of times so there is a risk of the tattoo site becoming infected. To reduce this risk you should use an antibacterial soap twice a day until the tattoo has healed.

* STIs. As with body piercing, diseases such as hepatitis B and C and HIV can be transmitted during tattooing if instruments have not been properly sterilised. Professional tattoo and piercing studios are usually well aware of these health risks and always sterilise their equipment after every session.

* Unwanted tattoo. You could end up regretting ever having a tattoo – either straightaway or years later, when your scene has changed – especially if you don't think it through.

Tattoo removal

Treatments to remove a tattoo take time, are costly and can lead to complications. They are unlikely to be performed on the NHS as it is seen as a cosmetic procedure. The best treatment to remove a tattoo that is currently available is by laser therapy. This is where pulses of specific wavelengths of light are beamed onto the tattoo to break up the pigment. The surrounding skin does not absorb the light and so remains unaffected. It is not particularly painful and so doesn't usually require an anaesthetic – most people describe the sensation as being like a rubber band snapping against their skin. But if you have a low threshold for pain then an anaesthetic cream can be used.

The procedure usually takes a number of sessions. How well the treatment works and how many sessions you need depends on the age, size and colour of the tattoo you want removed. The pigments used in black tattoos absorb a wider range of light wavelengths than coloured ones and so are said to be easier to remove. Thankfully, complications with laser treatment are generally minor and rare. But you can experience problems, such as the tattooed area being paler than the surrounding skin, infection of the tattoo site, and even some scarring. Very rarely, a raised or thickened scar can appear three to six months after the tattoo is removed. Although effective in most cases, laser therapy doesn't work completely for every tattoo, so you may be left with some pigment.

Other treatments available for the removal of tattoos are not as effective as laser therapy because they are more likely to cause scarring and so can't be recommended. One method is dermabrasion where your skin is 'abraded' – basically sanded down – to remove the surface and middle layers of skin, and hence the tattoo as well. Another method is surgery, but this leaves a scar and is only possible for small tattoos.

Another common method for hiding an unwanted tattoo (especially the name of an ex-boyfriend) is to cover it over with another design!

KEY POINTS

* Your skin is highly sensitive because it contains millions of nerve endings.
* 1 in 3 gay guys has a piercing – the most common is in the ear.
* 1 in 20 gay guys has some part of their genitalia pierced.
* The holes of piercings can take months to heal and so can be places where blood-borne infections such as hepatitis B and C and HIV can be picked up and passed on.
* Tattoos have become increasingly popular but don't have one done on impulse. A tattoo is difficult and expensive to remove if you get tired of it.

SIX

COCK

'I'm worried about my dick. All the guys I go with seem to be bigger than me. I'm only about 5 inches [12.5 cm] long when erect.' Simon, 22

Think of the amount of time and attention you spend on your penis, playing with it (or another guy's), keeping it looking good by clipping its hair, or having a piercing. Then there is the time you spend dreaming about penises, or looking at them in movies and magazines. Many gay men will admit to having cock on their minds a lot of the time!

The number one worry guys usually have with their penis is its size. If you start to believe what you see in magazines or porn films you'll soon become insecure about your own penis and disappointed when you find out that most guys you meet do not have a rock hard 8 or 9 inches. In reality, the problem that most men have about the size of their penis is in their own heads.

Understanding more about how your penis is built and how it works will help you get more from it. Knowing what's normal and what isn't will also show you when you have reason to be worried and when you can relax.

THE BASICS

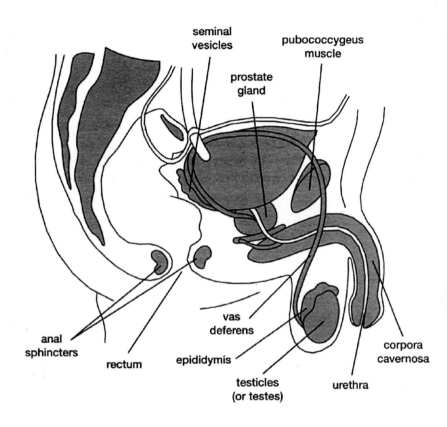

seminal vesicles

pubococcygeus muscle

prostate gland

anal sphincters

rectum

vas deferens

epididymis

testicles (or testes)

urethra

corpora cavernosa

Your penis has a very simple structure. It's made up of three basic parts – the root, the body and the head. This is all covered by a thin layer of skin.

Head

At the top of your penis is the head, or glans. This is a mass of tissue that comes from an extension of a cylinder of tissue called the corpus spongiosum, which makes up part of the body of the penis.

The head is supplied with thousands and thousands of nerve fibres, which makes it highly sensitive – especially the coronal ridge, or crown, that goes around the base of the glans. A very sensitive part is a small area called the fraenulum. This is where the foreskin attaches to the underside of your penis. It's so sensitive that many guys can orgasm just by being stimulated in that tiny area. But the fraenulum is a delicate area that contains an artery. So any slight tearing during sex can cause heavy bleeding. This usually happens when guys don't use enough lubricating gel during anal sex.

Body

The body, or shaft, of the penis is made up of three cylinders of spongy tissue. The two cylinders that lie side by side as you look down at your penis are called the corpora cavernosa. They are wrapped up in a strong membrane, the tunica albuginea. This membrane is really important because it is responsible for keeping your penis straight as it fills with blood when you get an erection. Any bending or break in the penis is most often caused by damage and scarring to this membrane. This usually happens when the penis is bent at an awkward angle during rougher sex (see page 187).

The third and smaller cylinder lies on the underside of the penis and is called the corpus spongiosum. Inside this cylinder is the urethra, which carries urine from your bladder and sperm and semen from the testicles and prostate when you ejaculate.

Root

The body of your penis runs deep inside the body and is anchored tightly into your pelvis by strong ligaments. This deep part of your penis is called, unsurprisingly, the root.

Skin

The whole penis is covered by a very thin layer of skin. This skin has no fat layer, no matter how large your penis, which is why you can usually see the veins running up the side.

The skin is attached quite loosely and this allows it to move freely up and down during sex. At the end of the penis, this skin is folded over to make the foreskin. The foreskin is supplied by many nerve fibres, making it super sensitive and pleasurable to touch and play with. The purpose of the foreskin is to protect the sensitive glans from damage or infection. But when you get an erection it has another function. As it slips behind the glans, it works like a weak tourniquet to trap blood in the glans. This makes it fatter and fuller and more sensitive. But of course that can only happen if you haven't been circumcised ('cut').

CIRCUMCISED OR UNCIRCUMCISED?

The classic picture of a penis that appears in films and magazine is often without a foreskin. When looking for sex, many men ask whether you're 'cut' (circumcised) or 'uncut' (uncircumcised), perhaps because they just prefer an uncircumcised penis or find a penis with a foreskin a turnoff. But for all the men who prefer an 'uncut dick' there are just as many who prefer one with the foreskin intact.

World-wide, about 1 in 2 men (50 per cent) is circumcised. In the UK, the figure among gay men is about 1 in 5 (20 per cent).[1] In some cultures, the foreskin is removed for religious reasons, usually during infancy or childhood. In other cultures it may be done for reasons of hygiene.

Sometimes a circumcision is necessary for medical reasons. The most common reasons are because of repeated infections of the foreskin (balanitis, see page 185) or because the foreskin is so tight that it cannot draw back over the head of the penis (phimosis, see page 186). This is a simple operation in childhood and is still pretty routine even for an adult, although there are risks (see below). It is normally carried out under a local anaesthetic. You will need stitches and must abstain from sex for up to a month until the wound has healed.

Some guys think about having a circumcision for purely cosmetic reasons. If you are considering this I would definitely advise you to think twice. Even though circumcision is a straightforward operation there is a slight risk of infection and heavy bleeding. It's also possible to take too much or too little away, so you could be left with an odd-looking penis. Following circumcision, the skin on the glans is permanently exposed and this can lead to a reduction in sensitivity and so make sex less pleasurable.

A foreskin – for those who have one! – can add a lot to your sex life. It is a very sensitive area and one that guys tend to forget about, thinking that they should be concentrating on the head of the penis. Some guys like to have the foreskin pierced, or to attach clamps or weights to it. These are all good reasons to keep your hood intact!

Getting it back – foreskin restoration

Some guys who have been cut wish they had a foreskin – usually for cosmetic reasons, as they see an 'uncut cock' as more natural and more normal. But there are lots of other reasons. They may feel they were circumcised against their will or want the extra sensitivity that the foreskin can provide.

Some men go to great lengths to get their foreskin back. Stretching techniques – with tape, weights or straps – are most often used. These gradually stretch what foreskin you have and can take years. Some private clinics offer 'quick-fix' surgical operations to restore your foreskin but, in general, they are not to be recommended. They have a low success rate and you could end up with a worse problem than when you started. Some websites have lots of information about this (see Further Information, Resources, Websites and Organisations, page 263).

Keeping it clean

Dead skin cells and the natural lubrication from the head of your penis can collect under your foreskin. This can all go to make that smelly, white, cheesy material called smegma. It's unpleasant stuff and a complete turn-off. Urine and semen can also get trapped here and will add to this if not washed away, so it's important to keep yourself clean. Also the area under the foreskin is damp and airless, so it makes an ideal environment for bacteria and fungi to feed and breed on this debris, leading to an infection.

How to keep clean

Many guys think that they need to wash the head of their penis as if they're washing the dishes. All you need to do is to draw the skin back from the head and wash around with water. Using soap can cause inflammation and a discharge if soapy water gets inside your urethra. Washing more gently but more frequently is a better idea.

Always gently pull back your foreskin when you urinate and wipe yourself dry when you're done and before you pull it forward again. This stops urine collecting under your foreskin and so keeping the area damp.

ARE YOU A SIZE QUEEN?

Every gay man looks around the beach imagining what might be hiding inside a pair of Speedos, or nudges his mates when a guy with a seemingly large member walks past. Many men – and not only gay men – judge themselves and others on the size of their cocks. Guys want big ones because size has come to indicate manliness and virility – even though this is just not true!

In reality, we all know that penises come in all shapes and sizes, and not every guy is hung like a horse. If you believe otherwise then you're setting yourself up for disappointment – not only in yourself, but also in the majority of guys out there!

Of course, gay men have a special interest in other men's cocks, so it's not surprising that issues of size are often paramount in a gay guy's mind. But let's get some facts straight. There are lots of different figures, but the following figures come from the guidelines set out for surgeons who carry out penis enlargement (and they should know!):[2]

* The average penis, when erect, is about 5.9 inches (14 cm) long.
* Over 60 per cent (around 2 in 3) of men have a penis that measures between 5.1 inches (12.75 cm) and 6.2 inches (15.5 cm).
* The average girth – around the thickest part – is just under 5 inches (12.5 cm).
* Around 75 per cent (3 in 4) of guys have a girth of between 4.5 inches (11.5 cm) and 5.5 inches (13.75 cm).

The size of your penis when you are twenty is the size it will be when you are fifty, so although your body gets smaller as you get older your penis stays the same size.

You can't always predict the size of an erect penis based on its size in the soft (flaccid) state. But a rule of thumb is that a small penis usually undergoes a proportionately bigger change in size when it becomes erect ('growers') compared to one that is long in the flaccid state, which generally doesn't always get much longer when hard ('showers'). For those with a small penis, it's unfortunate that it's the big penis that gets noticed in the changing room!

If you are average size or under, remember that most guys are not size queens and many guys actually prefer a smaller penis – it's easier to fit into the mouth and arse.

MAKING THE MOST OF WHAT YOU HAVE

There are lots of ways in which to show yourself in the best possible light – or to put it another way, make yourself look bigger than you actually are!

Clipping the pubic hairs short around the base of your penis is the most popular way because it exposes more of your penis. Many guys shave off their pubes entirely, as this exposes the whole of the penis, rather than leaving half of it hidden away in a mass of curls. But be careful when you do this – it's very easy to nick your skin, causing bleeding and the possibility of infection. For tips on clipping and shaving, see page 62.

MEASURING STRAIGHT

How many guys do you see describing themselves as large or extra large? In fact, the way many men measure themselves is wrong – either they're not giving themselves the length they deserve, or they're giving themselves a little extra. To measure your maximum penis length correctly you need to be standing and have an erection. Push your penis away from your body so that it's level (parallel) with the floor. Using a ruler, measure from your pubic bone (just above the base of your penis) to the very end.

'I'M TOO SMALL' – THE TRUTH ABOUT SURGERY

For most men, the idea that they have a small penis is in their heads and not their pants. There have been studies that show that most men who think they have a small cock in fact have a normal-size one, but just overestimate what normal is.[3] Internet sites and cosmetic clinics can add to these insecurities when most guys have nothing to worry about. Remember that even a small penis works perfectly well. Anyway, reputable surgeons won't operate unless you're less than 3 inches (7.5 cm) when hard.[4]

If you are over-conscious about your size and considering surgery, think again. Ask yourself why you're thinking of it. Did you start to feel insecure after someone made a comment about you or are you only judging yourself to be small?

You may be worried that you can't satisfy your partner. This is unlikely to be true as the size of your penis is only a part of your sex life, and it is far easier to change and improve your technique and add some extra fun and games to your sex life than having an operation. Also, you need to consider that if your partner is only interested in the size of your dick whether you should be with him at all.

Worries about size can be a sign of being unhappy about yourself in another way. Just as some guys might worry about the size of their pecs, others focus on their penis and feel that if only it were a couple of centimetres bigger then everything would be okay. But this is rarely true. Talking to a trained counsellor can help resolve issues like this.

Whatever your reasons for considering surgery, you will be putting a lot on the line. Despite what all the advertising may say, there is no very safe, easy method to increase what you have. In addition, many guys who subject themselves to the knife are not happy with the results.

There are lots of non-surgical gadgets on the market that can help you to reach your maximum. They are generally safe and so I'd encourage you to try these before resorting to surgery. Vacuum pumps and penile or tension ('cock') rings are the most commonly used devices. Vacuum pumps draw extra blood into your penis, and then a cock ring keeps it there. This gives you a bit extra and keeps you harder for longer.

Increasing length and width

Surgery to lengthen the penis involves cutting the ligaments that attach the root of the penis to the pubic bone. This is called the Bihari procedure and can release several centimetres of the penis that is normally hidden inside your lower abdomen by letting more of it hang away from your body. But the risk of this operation is that when you become aroused you can't get your penis to go fully erect. It may stick out at right-angles or even hang down.

Operations to increase the girth usually involve collecting fat from other parts of your body and injecting it under the skin along the shaft of your penis. However, the results can be less than desired. You may end up with a penis that feels lumpy and can look very odd and unappealing. The head of the penis can't be made any bigger so it will look out of proportion. You can end up with what looks like a tiny head on a fattened shaft.

GETTING AN ERECTION

Everyone knows that the penis gets hard because it fills with blood. But it's not just a simple matter of hydraulics (although many men wish sometimes it was as easy as flipping a switch) but a complex mix of mind and emotions – blood vessels and nerves all working together.

The usual state of a man's penis is soft (flaccid). That's because the spongy cylinders of tissue described earlier contain little blood. But when you get turned on through sexual thoughts, images or the cute guy who's just passed you in the street, messages are sent from your brain to the penis via the parasympathetic nerves. These nerves stimulate the release of chemicals such as nitric oxide, which make the blood vessels that supply your penis widen (dilate). More blood is let into your penis, thereby filling the spongy tissues. As you get erect, the valves in the veins that normally let blood leave your penis become closed, keeping blood trapped inside so you become harder and more erect. As you get more aroused the blood also makes the skin of your scrotum tighter and darker and your testicles become more compact and closer to your body.

You can see that it is a complicated process and so not surprising that about 1 in 10 men (10 per cent) will have erection problems at some time in his life. You may have problems getting an erection or keeping it long enough to enjoy sex. Emotional problems, damaged blood vessels or nerves, or low hormone levels can all be a cause. But there are lots of treatments to help with erection problems. For more about the causes and treatment of erection troubles, see page 189.

BENDS AND BREAKS

About 1 in 4 of all penises (25 per cent) bends in one direction or another – to one side, say, or up or down. If it doesn't cause pain or interfere with your sex life then you have nothing to worry about. But it could be a sign of a condition called Peyronie's disease. For more about that, see page 187.

KEY POINTS

* Your penis is made up of three cylinders of spongy tissue that fill with blood to give you an erection.
* Most men have a normal-size penis. Most men who worry that they're small overestimate what is normal.
* Keep the head of your penis clean. If you are uncircumcised, this means pulling back your foreskin and washing with water. Keep the area dry.
* Don't have surgery to enlarge your cock or remove your foreskin for purely cosmetic reasons.

SEVEN

BALLS

Your testicles, or balls, are the structures where millions of sperm and the male hormone testosterone are made. Many gay men don't care whether they're fertile or not, but they are interested in how much or how little semen ('cum') they produce. The hormone testosterone is in charge of giving you the shape and appearance of a man. It also governs your sex drive, so it's an important hormone. For many men, the testicles are also havens of sexual pleasure. Gentle tugs can heighten or delay orgasm and just playing with a guy's testicles may bring him to orgasm.

Naturally, your testicles are treasured possessions, hence all the jokes about them being 'crown jewels'. But, as with all body parts, things can go wrong. Most problems are not serious. Some however, such as testicular cancer, can be, especially if you don't catch it early on. So it's important to know about your testicles, how they work and what they normally feel like, so you can tell when there is a problem.

THE BASICS

As you know, your two testicles hang outside your body. This is so that they are kept at a lower temperature than the rest of your body – in fact, about 3°C cooler. This lower temperature is needed to optimise sperm production and explains why squeezing them into tight jeans, where they may overheat, can sometimes cause fertility problems.

Many men worry that one testicle is lower than the other or that they are not exactly the same size. But be reassured, this is perfectly normal. In most guys it is the left one that hangs lower and is slightly bigger than the right.

Each 'ball' is made up of a testicle, epididymis and vas deferens all held inside a sac, or bag, of skin called the scrotum.

Testicles

Testicle size varies from man to man but in most cases it is about the size of a walnut. Having bigger balls doesn't mean that you are more fertile, or have a greater sex drive, or that you make more semen. The main function of the testicles is to make sperm and the hormone testosterone. It is this hormone that turns boys into men (by triggering development of the sexual organs before birth, and the growth of facial, pubic and body hair, deepening of the voice, and development of the sex drive and mature sex organs at puberty). It also boosts muscle development, which is why some guys inject high doses of synthetic anabolic steroids to bulk themselves up.

Epididymis

Within your scrotum and at the back of each testicle is a mass of soft tubing called the epididymis. Each mass is, in fact, a set of tiny tubes which connect to form one tightly coiled tube that, if unravelled, would measure about six metres! The immature sperm from the testicles collect inside these coils and mature, developing the ability to propel themselves.

Vas deferens

Out from the coils of your epididymis runs a thick walled pipe called the vas deferens. Your sperm travel through this tube when you ejaculate, a journey of about 45 cm in most guys. The vas runs from your epididymis, up through your groin, deep into your pelvis and then along the outside of your bladder and finally into your prostate gland, connecting with the seminal glands on the way. These are the glands that add a sugary fluid, called seminal fluid, to the sperm. This feeds the sperm and starts them swimming. When you ejaculate, the semen is forced into the urethra, just after it leaves the bladder, and out of the body by a series of muscular contractions. (Semen is the name given to the mixture of sperm and seminal fluid.)

It takes around 100 days to make a sperm, from immature sperm to mature one:

* 74 days of growth within the testis.
* 20 days to pass through the epididymis.
* 6 days travelling through the vas deferens before ejaculation.

EJACULATION AND ORGASM

Ejaculation is when semen, containing your sperm, shoots out of your penis. An orgasm is the wave of pleasure you get when you ejaculate. Men can orgasm after as little as two to three minutes of sexual stimulation, but usually learn to delay this in order to extend their pleasure and that of their partner. The signs that your orgasm is on its way begin with a tightening of your balls. You'll also start to feel the stirrings of a deep sense of pleasure in your groin. Your blood pressure and heart rate go up, and blood rushes to the surface of the skin, making you feel warm. As you approach orgasm, you'll feel intense waves of muscular contractions from the vas deferens, pumping the semen into the urethra. This is followed by contractions of the prostate and urethra that pump semen down the urethra and out of your penis in a series of spurts that steadily diminish in force and frequency.

Once you have climaxed, your penis returns to its usual soft state. This is because the brain switches off the nerve impulses to the blood vessels in your penis and so the valves open and the blood drains away. Depending on lots of factors, such as your age and how turned on you are, it may be anything from minutes to hours before you can get hard again.

Scrotum

Your testicles are held inside a sac of skin called the scrotum. If you look carefully down the centre of your scrotum you'll see a slightly raised ridge where each half of your pouch is joined. This ridge is supplied with thousands of nerve endings, making it very sensitive – for many men it can be a focus of sex play and pleasure.

The skin of the scrotum is also wrinkled because of layers of muscles under the skin. These can make the skin loose and so give off heat to cool the testicle when you're hot, or contract and so bring the testicles close to the body to protect them and keep them warmer. One of these muscles is called the cremaster muscle and is responsible for your cremasteric reflex. That's where your testicles are pulled up tightly towards the body. It happens not only when you're cold or turned on but also when you're scared, as a primitive way of protecting your testicles from injury.

TIPS ON CLIPPING AND SHAVING

Many gay guys prefer a clean and tidy bush, bald scrotum and smooth butt. But, from a medical view, genital shaving can be hazardous as it can cause irritation or infection. It's also easy to cut the skin, which can bleed profusely.

If you are going to shave then start by carefully trimming the long hairs with clippers or scissors and then have a long bath to soften your skin. Next, put lots of moisturising shaving cream on the area you are going to shave and leave for five minutes. With a fresh blade shave with the grain of your hair and then make a second pass against the grain. Use a fresh blade with each new area you're shaving, or as soon as you feel the razor start to drag. Once you've finished, pat on some alcohol-free shaving lotion. To avoid irritation, aim to exfoliate and wash the area daily. Talc also helps to keep the skin dry and prevents itching.

A downside of shaving is that it can cause inflammation of the hair follicles – at the base of each hair. This condition, called folliculitis, is caused by infection with the bacterium *Staphylococcus aureus*, resulting in small pus-filled red spots. They should not be confused with boils, which are larger and generally only occur singly. Usually folliculitis does not require treatment and the condition settles over a week or so, but sometimes antibiotics are needed if the infection is severe. To prevent this infection always use fresh razor blades, wash with an antiseptic soap and dry with clean towels.

Alternatively, you can use hair-remover (depilatory) creams. Many guys especially prefer to use these for the anal area. They also stop your hair growing back so fast. Choose depilatory creams that say they are intended for the 'bikini' area. It's a good idea to test the cream on a small area of skin first. If that's okay, follow the instructions carefully. Don't leave the cream on too long or it will burn the skin.

Generally I'd avoid waxing or sugaring your scrotum – although 'back, crack and sack' is popular – unless you get thrills from pain.

Laser hair removal is a way to get rid of unwanted hair for longer, sometimes permanently. This involves shining special wavelengths of light onto your skin. The light penetrates to about two millimetres below the surface to reach the hair roots themselves, heating them up and destroying them. But the light can only destroy the roots where they are actually growing, and so not all your unwanted hair can be destroyed at once. You usually need a course of treatments.

As the light is absorbed by melanin (the pigment in the skin), it works better for light skinned and dark haired people. If you're dark skinned more light is absorbed, which can make your skin go darker or lighter – although this is not usually permanent. You can have laser treatment on any area of the body but treating your penis and anal area is difficult and can be painful.

Other methods that work for permanent hair removal include flash light therapy and electrolysis. With electrolysis, in which individual hairs are removed with a short burst of electricity, permanent hair removal can take a lot longer. Bear in mind that new hair follicles form as you get older so although you'll get a buff body at twenty-four you'll need to have more treatments as the years go by.

CHECKING YOURSELF – OR HIM – OUT

It's important that you know what your balls normally feel like so you can spot any problems as early as possible. The sooner you find out that there is anything wrong with your testicles the better.

Cancer of the testicles is the most common cancer of guys age 15–35 and can be cured if diagnosed early. If you do notice anything different, such as lumps or swellings, or you're not sure whether anything feels different, always see your GP for a check-up – and don't hang about!

It's best to check yourself, or your partner, when your scrotum is relaxed and loose – after a shower or bath, for example. That way it's easier to feel the testicles inside.

Using your thumb and forefinger you should feel all around each testicle. It should be smooth and oval-shaped. Check for lumps and swellings, which can be a sign of cancer (see page 207).

At the back of each ball is the epididymis. This will feel like soft coils of tubes and can be tender, so don't squeeze it hard! Common lumps here are called epididymal cysts. These are not cancers, but just fluid-filled sacs (see page 209). If your epididymis feels very sore when you touch it then you could have an infection (see page 205).

Finally, you should be able to feel the spermatic cord running from the top of your epididymis and up into your groin. This contains all the blood vessels and nerves, as well as the vas deferens.

SEMEN ('CUM')

Semen, also known as 'come' or 'cum', is the fluid that spurts out of your penis when you ejaculate. It is mostly liquid but it can also contain from 30 million to 140 million sperm. In total, you'll usually shoot about 2.7 to 3.4 mls, or half a teaspoonful, but the amount does vary.

The colour of semen is usually off-white, but can vary from yellowish to white or even clear. If there are ever traces of blood in your semen this can be a sign of a prostate infection (see page 201) so needs to be checked. However, traces or flecks of blood in the semen can also come from tiny blood vessels in your prostate which burst under the force of your orgasm. If it does not clear up in a day or two you should get medical attention.

Semen contains potassium and usually tastes slightly salty. But the flavour varies from one man to the next. Some foods affect how semen tastes, just as some foods make urine smell odd. For example, asparagus makes for an unpleasant taste whereas a diet rich in meat and fish is claimed to produce a smoother, more buttery flavour.

Shooting more and shooting further

The amount, quality and consistency of semen can vary substantially from man to man and even from ejaculation to ejaculation. If you want to produce a porn-show-style ejaculation try the following:

* Keep hydrated – semen is mostly water.
* Stick to a balanced diet, which includes fats. Being on a low-fat diet could reduce production because dietary fats are needed for testosterone production.
* Boost the volume. Make sure the only stuff to come out of your penis for a couple of days is pee. If you don't ejaculate for a few days, it will mean that when you do shoot you'll shoot a bigger load.
* Prime the pump. Masturbate a few hours before sex, but stop before you ejaculate. You'll produce more semen so that when you finally cum there will be an extra helping!
* Hold back for a better finale. The amount you spurt also depends on how aroused you are.

'I am 32 years old and have noticed that I don't shoot as far as I used to. It used to be a big turn on for me to shoot over guys but now I just seem to dribble out! Not much of a finale.' Dom, 32

Pelvic floor exercises

If you want to ejaculate further, you need to strengthen the muscles that help drive your ejaculation – the ones you squeeze to stop peeing. Pelvic floor or Kegel exercises (named after Dr Kegel, who invented them) help strengthen the muscles of the pelvic floor. These muscles – especially the pubococcygeus – are part of a network of muscles that support the organs in your lower abdomen, such as your bladder and rectum. They also play a role in controlling your bowels and bladder. Strong pelvic floor muscles can also give you a firmer erection, delay ejaculation, help give you more intense orgasms, ejaculate further, and keep your anal muscles in good shape and so able to squeeze more firmly on a penis inside you.

You can easily find these muscles by trying to stop urinating in mid flow and by tensing your anus, or by sticking a finger (or someone else's) in your anus and try squeezing on it. It's not like tensing your butt, abs or thighs – it's a squeezing and lifting feeling. And remember to breathe!

Once you get used to finding the pelvic floor muscles, there are lots of ways to do Kegels – here are a couple to choose from:

* Tighten and hold the muscles for 5–10 seconds, pause for 10 seconds and squeeze again. Do up to about ten squeezes every day and try to increase how long you hold for.
* Squeeze and relax over and over again. Aim for a couple of minutes or fifty squeezes to start, but you can work up to 20 minutes or a couple of hundred squeezes.

The great thing about Kegels is that you can do them anywhere and no one will know you're doing them. Like all muscle training, don't expect immediate results, but with time you will notice the difference.

KEY POINTS

* Your testicles, or balls, are where millions of sperm and the hormone testosterone are made.
* When you orgasm your balls become tight and are pulled up close to your body. This also happens when you're cold or afraid as a way of keeping the testicles warm or protecting them from possible harm.
* Shaving your testicles can be risky – you can cut yourself and the hair follicles can get infected. If you do shave, use clean razor blades and antibacterial soap.
* An alternative is depilatory creams, but these may irritate the skin.
* Examine your testicles regularly for lumps. See your GP at once if you feel any.
* If you want to shoot a bigger load and shoot it further, avoid ejaculating for a few days, keep fully hydrated and practise Kegel exercises.

EIGHT

ARSE

Why is it important to know about your arse? Well, it can be a source of great sexual pleasure and so the more you know the greater your chances of having more fun. But it can also be a source of pain. The arse is a delicate area and can be easily damaged. However, it can be hard to learn about – most obviously because a great deal of it is hidden away and difficult to see.

Understanding this part of your anatomy will make sex more pleasurable for yourself and for your partner. This knowledge will also help you to have safer sex and know when things aren't right.

THE BASICS

'Arse' is a pretty general word that guys use to describe a lot of different things. It's a word that some use to describe the big buttock muscles – the gluteus maximus – that give the butt its bubble shape (or not, as the case may be!). It can also mean your anus (or arsehole), the opening made up of rings of muscle through which you pass faeces. Before I describe it, it's a good idea to start further up the digestive tract so that you know what comes higher up.

The anus is the very end of what is called your digestive or gastro-intestinal (GI) tract, a system of tubes and other organs that extracts all the nutrients from the food you eat. When you swallow food it goes down a food pipe, called the oesophagus, into your stomach. This is a hollow J-shaped organ that plays a part in the digestion of food by mixing it with enzymes and churning it up.

After spending a few hours in your stomach, the now liquid food passes into your small intestine. The tubes of the small intestine are just 2.5 cm across but run for over 6 m. As the liquid food passes along these tubes, nutrients and fluid are taken out and absorbed into your body.

The end of the small intestine connects with a larger tube called the large intestine, or colon, which goes up, across and down your abdomen. More water is taken out of your food as it passes through the large intestine, and it slowly becomes more solid. Eventually, all that is left is mostly unwanted waste, called faeces.

The last part of the large intestine is made up of the sigmoid colon and rectum. They are separated by a ring of muscle, or sphincter, that acts as a valve to stop the waste matter from going any further. The sigmoid colon allows faeces to build up and then the sphincter relaxes and faeces passes into the rectum.

The rectum, anal canal and anus

The rectum is an S-shaped and fairly spacious tube 10–13 cm (about 4–5 in) long. It is supported by muscles that contract in a rhythmic way when you open your bowels. The walls of the rectum are very thin and contain lots of blood vessels, but few nerve endings, so you have little sensation there. In fact, the rectum is only sensitive to stretch. It is easily damaged through rough sex, use of toys, or fisting, and is an area where sexually transmitted infections (STIs) and viruses, such as HIV, can readily enter the body because the lining is naturally very absorbent – just like a sponge. Because it is so absorbent some guys insert recreational drugs this way, and prescription medications can also be given via the rectum as special large tablets called suppositories.

The lower part of the rectum tilts forwards towards your navel. It then curves sharply backwards, in the opposite direction, towards your backbone. The curve is caused by a muscle, called the puborectalis muscle, that swings around this part of the rectum to form the puborectal sling, and keeps the rectum bent at almost 90 degrees. This serves to keep any faeces or gas in the upper rectum, but it can relax and so let the rectum almost straighten out completely when you empty your bowels to let the faeces pass down and out.

It's important to know about this curve because it means you, or your partner, need to angle your penis when you insert it into the anus. Go slowly, to nudge the muscular sling out of the way and so let the rectum straighten, or adopt positions such as squatting that automatically straighten it out. If you don't do this, it is one of the main reasons why anal sex can be so painful.

The puborectalis muscle is just one of many muscles that form what's called your pelvic floor. This supports your bladder and other internal organs and stops them slipping down into your pelvis. These are the muscles that you can tense and so train to become stronger to give you firmer erections, more pleasurable orgasms, and to shoot your load further – often called pelvic floor or Kegel exercises (see page 65).

Below your rectum there is a pair of doughnut-shaped sphincter muscles, which make up your anus. They form a short tube, 2.5–4 cm (about 1–1½ in) long, called the anal canal, that is deeply folded and lined with cushions of tissue filled with delicate blood vessels. These blood vessels can become swollen and form piles (haemorrhoids, see page 212), that can then bleed when you go to the toilet. Right at the end of the rectum are glands that produce anal mucus, which lubricates the canal to help faeces pass through more easily.

Along with the muscular rectal sling described above, the two anal sphincters control both 'exit and entry'. But they have important differences that you need to know about.

The external sphincter holds the anal canal in shape. It is a voluntary muscle, just like the muscles of the arms, legs and face, that you can consciously move, and so this means that you have some control over it. You can relax it by straining slightly, as if you wanted to open your bowels, or clench it, as if you're trying to stop yourself going to the toilet or farting.

The internal sphincter is a different type of muscle, called an involuntary muscle. This means that you have less direct control over it because it is controlled by the part of your nervous system that works automatically.

Knowing about your anal sphincters is very important when it comes to anal sex. Although both muscles have the ability to stretch very wide, the internal sphincter can't tell the difference between faeces or a penis so it naturally tenses up when it detects anything inside. It will relax to let the faeces out, or a penis in, but you need to wait for up to 30 seconds to let this happen. Forcing a penis or a toy into the anus will cause the internal sphincter to go into spasm – which is very painful. (To learn more about how to prevent this happening in anal sex, see page 112.)

KEEPING CLEAN

'My problem is that I can never clear my bowel out enough to have sex. I even try anti-diarrhoea tablets on the day to firm myself up.' John, 32

Some men who enjoy anal sex worry at times about 'being dirty'. But it is natural that when you're having anal sex there's going to be some faeces about so you need to get used to that idea. If you're doing the penetration always wear a condom to protect yourself against the bacteria and other bugs that are in faeces, and to avoid contracting and/or transmitting an STI.

Gently wiping outside of your anus is basic hygiene and shows consideration for your partner. Generally speaking, the rectum only contains faeces when your bowels are full, so evacuating your bowels before sex is usually all that's needed to reduce the chance of any mess. Having a good diet that is full of fibre and drinking plenty of water should make your bowel movements softer and more bulky so that they pass more easily and are less likely to leave any residue in the rectum.

Men who want to be as clean as possible use enemas or douches. An enema involves using a water bottle with a long tube attached to insert up to half a litre (about a pint) of warm water into the rectum. You will be able to hold this water inside by clenching your buttock muscles and anal sphincter. After five minutes or so, you let the water out and it takes the faeces out with it.

Anal douching is similar but usually uses smaller quantities of water and so doesn't clean so far up the rectum. Some guys use ear syringes or ball douches to douche with. These, like enemas, are available in different sizes and can be bought from many chemists or sex shops and also on-line. (Some come ready-filled with perfumes, or medication to prevent constipation, and so must be emptied first.)

In general, a light douche is all that is necessary. Only ever use plain, clean water and it's best to ensure that it is as close to body temperature as possible. Some douches can be attached to showers but these are potentially harmful and should be avoided as you can't control the force of the water or the temperature.

Some men get too carried away with trying to be clean. Enemas and douches can irritate and even damage the lining of the rectum – especially if you use disinfectants or antiseptics. This can make it easier for bacterial infections and viruses, such as HIV, to pass through the lining of the rectum into your bloodstream. Using them regularly can also cause chronic constipation, and you may end up being unable to open your bowels without using a douche or laxative.

Deep douching is no more effective than a light douche, and there is the risk that some of the liquid you insert may not come out before you have sex. Later on, a thrusting penis inside you can make your colon contract and force out all the residue. You can end up in a bigger mess than if you hadn't used a douche in the first place.

The prostate

While the look of the arse might be what turns you on, all the action is on the inside. And the site of all the action is the prostate gland. Many gay men don't know about their prostate – or where it is. But the prostate is a major sexual pleasure centre – the male 'G spot' – so locating and learning about it is well worth the effort.

You can't see the prostate gland but you can feel it by inserting a finger about 4–8 cm (1½–3 in) inside the anus and towards the belly button. It is not actually inside your rectum. It sits at the base of your penis, just under the bladder, right next to the wall of the rectum. It is a doughnut-shaped gland about the size of a walnut that encircles part of the urethra at the point where the tube leaves the bladder and connects to the vas deferens.

The prostate produces fluid that helps to make semen. The prostate becomes enlarged in later life and because it also surrounds the urethra it can restrict or even block the flow of urine.

The prostate is important in sex because it contains lots of nerve fibres and gives a pleasurable sensation when it is stimulated through fingering or from anal sex. It can also make your orgasms more intense. To learn more about how to find and stimulate your prostate see page 113.

KEY POINTS

* Your rectum is not a straight tube but S-shaped.

* The lower part bends around a sling of muscle called the puborectal sling that helps prevent faeces or wind escaping until you open your bowels, when it moves out of the way to let the rectum straighten.

* Your anus is made up of a pair of anal sphincter muscles that control entry and exit from your rectum. You can relax the outer one at will, but the inner one is an involuntary muscle, which means you can't control it. However, it relaxes automatically after a few seconds.

* Enemas and heavy douching can irritate the lining of your rectum.

* Light douching with an ear syringe is usually all that is necessary to keep the anus and rectum clean for anal sex.

* The prostate gland sits at the base of your penis and can be felt a few centimetres inside your rectum, towards your belly button.

* The prostate makes fluid that mixes with your sperm to make semen.

PART III
SEX

NINE

LET'S TALK ABOUT SEX

'For me, sex can be a quick shag with someone I've just picked up, or a night with my boyfriend where we take our time. Both are just different types of sex for me – one is more about lust and the other is more about really caring and sharing with someone.' Greg, 25

Sex plays a big role in most gay men's lives. Besides being pleasurable, having (and bragging about) sex can be a way of confirming who you are. The beauty of sex is that it can mean so many different things. For some, sex can be quite impersonal – like a quick blow job in a club cubicle or a random pick-up where you get just what you want. At times like that it's simply about lust and feeling horny but can still be an intense emotional experience. At the other end of the spectrum, there is sex with someone that you feel totally connected with and who you care for or love. Sex then, while being just as hot, can also be about showing deeper feelings and about communicating your love. And there are all shades of sex between.

'I haven't had sex yet – or been fucked, anyway – but I have sucked a guy off. I have got one friend who says that he's done everything with loads of

guys and it makes me feel like a real loser. I suppose I'm basically a bit scared of sex and about how much it will hurt. I watch porn and just can't imagine that I've go to do what they do.' Isaac, 18

When it comes to what you do during sex there is no such thing as 'normal' in the gay world. For one guy, sex is sucking another guy off, for another it's about kisses and cuddles, and for others it's about being strung up in a sling. No one sex act defines what sex is. For a start, sex doesn't have to mean anal sex. In fact, many gay guys never have anal sex – it's just not for them. Gay men are lucky that they can enjoy a wide range of sex activities and have loads of sexual options. And it's natural to prefer one activity over another.

Most gay men get no gay sex education in school. Although there is sex educa-tion in general, because there is so much ground to cover regarding heterosexual issues, gay relationships often get forgotten. Many teachers are nervous about the subject and what they can and cannot teach – a hang-up from the now defunct Section 28 that prohibited local authorities from promoting homosexuality. But these factors are now being addressed in our schools and so things will change.

Although there is a lot of accurate information available on the web or from voluntary or charitable organisations, there is a lot of inaccurate information, too. Plus, many gay men get their ideas about gay sex from porn films and from the media in general. These images foster the impression that gay men are sex machines, always on the lookout for sex and permanently 'up for it'. Gay sex is always shown as involving wild, nightlong sessions with other men – guys who are also always hot, hung and hard. These images are great to fantasise about – and to watch – but portray an image of gay sex that is far from reality for most gay men. If you choose to believe it, this can leave you with feelings of inadequacy and anxiety over what kind of sex you feel you should be having and with how many people, especially if you are just starting out. You can then spend more time worrying than enjoying what you are doing.

It's true that some gay men have many partners and have lives based around sex. But that's not for everyone. Some gay men are not up for sex all of the time, and some do not want sex with anyone. Some guys prefer anonymous sex while other guys need a connection. Believing that you have to fit into a mould can leave you feeling out of place and worried that you're not 'normal'. It can also put you under pressure to have sex at times when you don't want to.

WHAT, WHEN AND HOW MANY?

There is some information about what kind of sex gay men have, and how many partners they have. Over the last few years, researchers have asked thousands of gay men across the UK about their sex habits. But it's worth bearing in mind that these were guys who were on the scene – they were found in bars, gay festivals and via the Internet – so these studies may not be true of all gay men, as many don't go to such events or places. This research found that:[1, 2, 3, 4, 5]

* 2 in 10 men (20 per cent) have one partner.
* 3 in 10 men (30 per cent) have two to four partners.
* 1 in 4 men (25 per cent) have five to twelve partners.
* 1 in 4 men (25 per cent) have more than thirteen partners.

These studies found that it is guys in their thirties who have the most partners. The average age for a first gay sexual experience is just over seventeen years old but the average age for anal sex is just over twenty years, usually with an older guy.

* 7 in 10 men (70 per cent) said they had anal sex in the last year (meaning 3 out of 10, or 30 per cent, did not).
* Over 9 in 10 men (95 per cent) had oral sex – both giving and receiving.
* Only 1 in 10 men (10 per cent) had fisted someone or been fisted himself, and a similar number had played with water sports.

These studies found that older men have more adventurous sex, probably because they are more confident with who they are and so want to explore it further. These results show that there is great variety in what gay men do and how many men they do it with.

What is great sex and how do I have it?

It's hard to say exactly what great sex is. I'd say that great sex is simply any type of sex that feels great at the time – both for you and the guy you're doing it with – and that you can also look back on as being great.

It's about feeling free to express your sexual side, to ask for what you want and to do what you want without feeling worried about how you're doing it or bad about what you're enjoying. It's not about how good you look or the size of your pecs! The guy who has the best sex will be the one who feels good about himself on the inside not necessarily the guy who looks the best on the outside.

NOT HAPPY WITH YOUR SEX LIFE?

In a survey,[6] about 3 in 10 gay men (30 per cent) say they are not happy with their sex life. The most common reason given by far is not having a relationship. But for 1 in 4 men (25 per cent) who aren't satisfied, lack of confidence is the main reason. For another 1 in 4 (25 per cent), the reason given was not having enough sex! Other reasons included worry about having safer sex, erection problems and concerns over a relationship.

It's also good to remember that no particular type of sex is better than any other. Every sexual experience has some kind of effect on you. So whatever type of sex you have, and for whatever reason you have it, the only rules you should try to follow are that you are doing it because you want to, that you won't regret it later, and that you do it safely. It is all too easy – especially if you are starting *out* – to have sex that you don't enjoy or feel comfortable with. You should only go as far as you want to and no one has the right to push you beyond your limits.

But there are a few practical considerations to having great sex. You may think these obvious but you'd be surprised that many guys give themselves a hard time when sex doesn't go well or when they don't perform as they think they should.

Technique: It's likely that you learnt your technique a little from magazines, books, the Internet, friends and a lot from experience. While many of these sources can give you an accurate grasp of how to have gay sex, a lot of what you see or that your friends talk about is pure fantasy. For many guys, sex just comes naturally but there are some sex facts to learn that will make it all a lot easier. Later in this chapter there are a few tips that you may find helpful.

State of body: If you're feeling tired or unwell, then no matter what your sexual partner does, you're not likely to have great sex.

State of mind: Not feeling right about the situation or being worried about something will affect your ability to relax and let go. Feeling confident and happy makes it more likely that you'll have a good sexual experience. Some gay men use drugs, either when they have sex or when they are looking for it. This may help to give you confidence but all drugs have their dangers (see page 230).

Fancying your partner: If you don't find your partner hot then you're not going to have great sex. It can take time to know what kind of guys turn you on. But with time you'll soon find out. There are occasions when this doesn't matter – you just want any cock or arse – but great sex will usually be when you find the whole person attractive.

Communication: Verbal and physical communication is probably one of the most important ingredients in your sex life. Communication is vital before you have sex, when you're talking with a cute guy about what he's into, and during sex, when you want him to do something for you or you don't like what he's doing. Unless you can communicate with your partner, it's likely that your sex will be less than ideal. It may seem embarrassing talking about sex, but I think you'll find that the more you feel able to talk about it the better the sex you'll have.

If you want adventurous, spontaneous sex that pushes the boundaries then you need to feel free enough to go there. Sex has been described as a mirror – if you don't feel free to give what you'd like to get then you won't receive it. So the tricks and positions you know for sex will always end up being about who you're doing it with and about the spark of attraction and chemistry between you. It's a two (or more) person thing.

Guilt and the gay guy

'My dad always wanted me to be like other boys. I always felt like I was disappointing him and it has always made me feel guilty about having feelings towards men. I think it really affected how I first started my sexual life – for ages I felt that what I wanted to do was just wrong and dirty.'
Rod, 28

Sex is not simple – although everyone thinks it should be. It can be a psychological minefield, especially between guys. Many of us have felt a level of guilt about being gay at some time or other, either about the fact that we desire other guys or about the kind of sex we want. So it's natural that if you have any negative feelings about your sexuality it will affect both the type of sex you have and your enjoyment of it. This can even work on a subconscious level, so you may not fully realise it. Even the most openly and sorted gay guy can still have these feelings.

This kind of guilt can be a reason why so many gay guys have quick, anonymous sex often under the influence of drink or drugs. Once the drugs have worn off it is still possible to feel bad about what you did or the fact that you desired it in the first place.

Being happy with who you are and what you like to do is central to enjoying a healthy sex life. You are entitled to have a full and enjoyable sex life and let no one tell you anything different! Guilt and shame should never stand in your way. It can take a long time to accept who you are and to realise that you should not feel guilty for being who you are or for having the kind of sex you want. But I hope that reading this book will help you to feel more confident about who you are and to enjoy your sexuality.

I believe that the more you know about sex and the more informed you are about how to do it safely, the greater your chances of having a good – or even great – sex life. Chapters 10, 11 and 12 will describe sex acts that range from the 'vanilla' (mild) to the 'hard core'. Finding out where you are on that scale and accepting what you enjoy will be your route to great sex. Remember that there is no 'normal' in sex and the route to a good sex life is accepting and letting yourself find your own sexual turn-ons.

SAFER SEX

Safer sex is all about trying to lower your chances of contracting sexually transmitted infections (STIs), especially HIV, while still having a full and enjoyable sex life. And so safer sex mainly focuses on using condoms for sex. If you have unsafe sex it usually means you don't use condoms to try to prevent the exchange of bodily fluids.

How much a condom reduces your risk of contracting an infection depends on the STI you are talking about. For example, wearing condoms for anal sex will greatly reduce the risk of HIV, as the virus is present in blood and semen, fluids that are easily exchanged during anal sex. Other STIs, for example herpes, warts or syphilis, are spread by close body contact and so a condom may not necessarily prevent infection. Detailed information about each infection and how to avoid getting it and passing it on is given in Chapter 13.

Safer sex is not only about condoms, however. It's also about the type of sex you have. Certain types of sex carry more risk of transmitting HIV than others and so it's up to you to decide how much risk you are happy to take. Kissing, frottage, massage, mutual masturbation, and oral sex with a condom are said to be low risk – because there is little or no exchange of bodily fluids. It is now clear that you can pick up the HIV virus through performing oral sex – that's when you suck his penis – on a man with HIV if he doesn't use a condom. Many men choose to take the risk and practise oral sex without a condom, while others have changed their habits and now do use one. The greatest risk of contracting and transmitting HIV is from unprotected anal sex or sharing sex toys.

Research shows that the more sexual partners you have the greater the risk that you'll pick up an STI. Perhaps one of the best ways to reduce your risk is by being able to talk to your partners about what you will and won't do – before you have sex. This makes it less likely that you'll practise risky sex – or unsafe sex – in the heat of the moment.

Other ways to reduce your risk of STIs are to:

★ Get tested routinely and often, perhaps every year if you're changing partners.
★ Get tested straight away if you suspect you have an infection, so you can get treated.
★ Avoid having sex until you have been given the all-clear. This prevents you passing on the infection to someone else.
★ Avoid using alcohol or drugs during sex, which can lower your inhibitions and cloud your judgement.

Men in monogamous relationships often want to stop using condoms. If both have had a full sexual health screening after at least three months of being together and are both clear from all infections then it is okay to stop using condoms. Three months is the minimum because it takes that long for HIV antibodies to show up in the blood. But you both have to be certain that neither one of you will play around, so this is a decision to be taken only after a lot of thought.

Some men have open relationships where they play around – always with condoms – but decide to stop using condoms at home. This is called 'fluid bonding' as a technique. Again, this kind of decision needs to be talked through carefully and requires a high level of trust in your partner.

Men in relationships where both partners are HIV positive should still continue to use condoms. If you don't you run the risk of contracting your partner's strain of HIV, which might be resistant to the anti-HIV drugs you are currently using. This is called 'superinfection'. If you are considering stopping using condoms or you have actually stopped then it's a good idea to discuss this with your HIV specialist. The specialist can evaluate your virus and your partner's to see how they compare and so estimate what the possible result could be if you stopped using condoms.

Condoms

Using condoms for sex is the best way that you can reduce the risk of contracting infection, so they deserve special attention. The better informed about them you are, the more likely you are to be happy to use them and to use them safely.

Condoms come in different shapes and sizes – and the first step is to find one that fits you properly and feels comfortable. Size differences in the girth can be up to 1.5 cm, so if you are using a condom of the wrong size it could be much too tight or too loose. This can also mean that the condom is more likely to split or fall off during sex. Smaller condoms, such as Pasante Trim or Mates Conform, are described on the packet as 'snug fit'. The most popular larger ones are Trojan Magnum XL and Pasante Large.

Condoms are available in a variety of materials. Most are made of latex, which is a type of rubber. It is possible to have an allergy to latex, in which case your penis might develop red blotches or feel sore after sex, but as most types are now hypoallergenic this is less likely. Some brands, such as one called Avanti, are made of polyurethane, which is a type of thin plastic. Some men prefer this condom because it is thinner and does not have a rubbery smell. Also you can use all types of lubricating gel ('lube') with it, even oil-based ones, because they don't damage polyurethane the way they do rubber (see below).

On the downside, polyurethane is more expensive and some men say they notice a little more noise! The third type of condom, which is quite new on the market, is made from a resin. One brand, called Unique, is made by Pasante. It is very thin and strong and can be used with any lubricant. It is rolled in a slightly different way and so looks different from the usual rolled condom. However, some men don't get on so well with this type of condom. It has no ring at the end to secure it in place and some say it can stick to the head of the penis and so be a little uncomfortable to take off.

Until recently, the message was that thicker or 'extra strong' condoms were safer for anal sex. But research shows that if used properly regular ones are just as safe. Never 'double up' in a bid to gain even better protection, as this can actually increase the risk of the condom splitting. There are lots of novelty condoms, too, but it's best to avoid these for anal intercourse, as they may not be so reliable.

Check the expiry date – condoms are more likely to split when old – and make sure that it has a 'CE' mark, which means that it has been checked and tested. Some guys have been known to wash condoms and reuse them – don't!

Lube

Along with condoms, lube is the other essential product for sex, as the anus does not produce enough natural lubrication for penetration. Without artificial lube, sex can be uncomfortable and can damage your rectum. It is also more dangerous because the condom is more likely to split. So use lube and lots of it for anal sex. There is usually some on condoms already but this is not enough. Not all lubes are the same, so you need to know which ones to use and which ones to avoid.

The right type: Water-based lube: Common types are Wet Stuff and Astroglide. Most well-known high street chemists sell own-brand lubes that are fine to use with all condoms but may dry out quickly, so you will need to keep the lube tube handy.

Silicone-based lube: Although more expensive, silicone-based lube, such as Eros Pjur, is more likely to last the whole session and you only need smaller amounts. It can also be used with sex toys and as a massage oil, but it can stain your sheets.

The wrong type: Anything oil-based, such as massage oil or baby oil, moisturiser, hand cream, oil, margarine and butter (you'd be surprised what some people reach for when they get going), can weaken most condoms, making them rot and split. The exception is Avanti condoms, as any kind of lube is okay with this type.

How to put on a condom

1 Open the packet carefully – don't use your teeth as this can rip the condom without you noticing. Some guys open a packet or two before they get down to sex to avoid any rush.

2 Start to unroll it a little on your finger, to make sure you know which way it goes on your penis – but no more than two turns. It should unroll easily, with the rolled ring of the condom on the outside. If it doesn't unroll easily it may be upside down.

3 Hold the tip to squeeze out the air and roll it all the way down to the base of your penis. If you're uncircumcised, remember to pull back your foreskin first.

Don't put lube inside the condom as the condom is more likely to slip off and also more likely to split. Once you've put the condom on, you can use as much lubrication as you like on the outside.

Now you're ready to go!

Condoms are good for about 45 minutes of anal sex – past that and you should change it for a new one. Every now and then, both of you should check to see that the condom is still in place. Of course, if you're having group sex then put on a new condom for each guy you have sex with.

If you've had anal sex, once you ejaculate, hold the base of the condom as you withdraw your penis. It's best to do this pretty soon after you cum, while you're still a little hard. This makes it less likely that the condom will slip off and spill the contents inside his anus. Dispose of it carefully. Wrap it in a tissue and throw it away – but remember it won't flush down the loo! If you're using it when cruising try to take it away with you, rather than leaving it lying around.

Condom failure

Condoms can split. The most common reasons are that the men didn't know how to use it properly, or used the wrong size, or used the same one for too long, or used saliva as a lubricant, or didn't use enough lubricant, or used the wrong type, which weakened the condom and made it tear.

It's always best to check the condom after use to make sure it's intact. If it's damaged, then talk this through with your partner. Remember, if you know he has HIV there are medications that can help to prevent you picking up the virus (see page 175).

THE FEMIDOM

Some guys use the female condom, which is sold under the brand name Femidom. This is a type of condom that is made to go inside the vagina, but it can be used inside the anus too. It has a small inner ring and a larger outer ring. It can either be used as an extra-baggy condom (in which case take the small ring out) or fitted inside the anus before you start to have sex (in which case leave the small ring in) so it is there ready when you decide to have anal sex.

Where to get condoms and lube

Condoms and lube are on sale almost everywhere nowadays, from high street chemists and sex shops to pubs and garages and on the Internet. Condoms are also available free from most genito-urinary medicine (GUM) clinics and family planning clinics. Also most gay pubs, clubs and saunas give them out, but don't rely on that – always have a couple of your own handy. They can be a little embarrassing to buy at first but remember that you are not alone; everyone has sex, so you should feel good about the fact that you are planning to have it too – especially as you're being responsible about it.

Some places only sell the most common brands and sizes, but if you buy online you have access to a wider variety and you can check out all the latest types and prices. (See Further Information, Resources, Websites and Organisations, page 263.)

UNSAFE SEX AND HIV

Research shows that up to 1 in 4 gay men (25 per cent) has at least one episode of unprotected anal sex a year with a casual partner who has a different HIV status to his own or whose HIV status is unknown to him.[7]

One survey, in 2005, showed that nearly 1 in 5 (20 per cent) who already had HIV had had unprotected anal sex with another HIV-positive man.[8]

The reasons why guys – no matter their HIV status – don't use condoms are complex. The following are comments on the subject:

'I didn't start out thinking I wouldn't use one but we were both a bit high and really into each other. I suppose my brain was just not switched on and we got carried away.' Paul, 24

'He didn't ask me to use one so I assumed he was positive, like I am.' Amrish, 25

'He just seemed like such a nice guy and I couldn't imagine that he had HIV – I mean, he has a responsible job and everything. He was also really hot – way out of my league, so I just felt I couldn't say no.' Sebastian, 30

'I lose my hard-on as soon as I put a condom on – every time – and without one I'm fine! And it just doesn't feel the same.' Rob, 30

Current treatments are much better than before, but HIV is still a serious illness that has a tremendous impact on your whole life. Protecting yourself and others is your responsibility – whether you are HIV negative or positive.

When you think through all the reasons guys give for not using condoms they don't really stack up. We all know that it is easy to get carried way when you're having sex – and especially if you've been drinking or taking drugs. Men who use Class A drugs are the least likely to use condoms for sex. If this applies to you then try talking about safer sex before you start out – don't leave it till you're both worked up. And have condoms to hand. If it becomes clear that things are heading towards penetration say, 'Can I get a condom?'

Assuming that someone is HIV positive or negative just because they didn't ask to use a condom is no way to run your sex life. Bear in mind that 1 in 3 men (33 per cent) with HIV doesn't know he has the virus so will assume he is negative. You can't tell someone's HIV status just by looking at them.

There is often a break in the flow while you get out a condom and put it on and many men find this a bit of a comedown. If you know that you lose your erection while you fit a condom then there are a few simple things that you can try. For example, use a penile ('cock') ring to keep you hard, or get your partner to play with you while you get ready, to sustain the excitement – or better still, get him to put it on for you. As mentioned before, you can also use a Femidom, which can be in place already so there is no delay in finding a condom and putting it on.

HIV and the law

Although the law is changing all the time, and so the situation is not very clear, some men have been prosecuted for passing on HIV to their partners. Those prosecuted so far have been heterosexual men, but cases involving gay men are in the pipeline. Currently, prosecution is based on the fact that the guy with HIV knew he was positive and didn't use condoms for sex. His partner was unaware of him having HIV – and he passed it on, whether on purpose or just through recklessness. So it is possible that if you are HIV positive and don't tell your partner or use condoms for sex and he gets infected, he could make a complaint to the police. It's also possible that the same thing could happen if you're HIV positive, your condom splits and you don't tell him so that he can get post-exposure prophylaxis (PEP).

There is a big debate on whether prosecuting someone for transmitting the virus will reduce rates of transmission or discourage men from having unsafe sex. Many agencies such as the Terrence Higgins Trust don't agree with the law as it stands. At present it is your choice whether or not you disclose your HIV status but bear in mind that safer sex is the responsibility of everyone. However, this is a new area of the law and one that everyone should keep an eye on. The Trust has a website that you can check out to keep up to date (see Further Information, Resources, Websites and Organisations, page 263).

KEY POINTS

* Film and media images and bad information about gay sex can make you feel inadequate about your own sex life. Don't believe the hype.

* Sex to you may be different from what sex means to someone else. There is no 'normal' sex in the gay world.

* Studies show that the number of partners that gay men have varies widely: 1 in 4 have had only one partner and the same proportion have had more than 13. The other 2 out of 4 fall somewhere between these two.

* Studies show that 7 in 10 men have anal sex, which means 3 in 10 do not.

* Better sex comes from being comfortable in your own skin and from having the freedom to express and ask for what you like.

* Using a condom can help prevent the spread of most STIs, including HIV.

* Latex condoms weaken and split if used with oil-based lube. Only use water-based lube or choose newer polyurethane condoms, such as Avanti, which are fine with all types of lube.

* If you know you have difficulty using condoms there are ways around the problem.

* The law is constantly changing, but if you are HIV positive and practise unsafe sex with an HIV negative man and he contracts the infection, you may be prosecuted.

TEN

THE NUTS, BOLTS (AND SCREWS) OF SEX

This section is about the sex acts that many gay men enjoy. With each act I'll describe what it is, a bit about how to do it, the health risks involved and how to enjoy it safely.

Sex is much more than technique, or a matter of ticking off each sex act on a list. But the sex acts described here are the basic building blocks of your sex life. How you put them together is for you to decide. You'll have favourites and there will be some that you won't enjoy. And what you like to do with one guy will be different from what you to do with others.

Now to the nuts and bolts (and screws) of sex – from foreplay to fucking and a whole lot between. If you're past these basics then you can jump straight to Chapter 12 – but every guy can benefit from being reminded about the health risks involved in their favourite activity.

FOREPLAY

'We normally dress up a little. I usually ask him to put on his Speedos because he has such a cute butt! Getting worked up together is the best part of sex for me.' Benjamin, 26

Foreplay is the time spent messing about before the action really begins. It's a time where you warm up, relax and get in the mood for sex. Some men are into it and want to spend as long as they can to work themselves up, while others are worked up enough already and just want to get on with the real action, without any foreplay.

What turns you on and puts you in the mood for sex is likely to be different from the next man and you can't always predict who will find what hot. Arousal usually starts with what you can see, but think about all your other senses, too, such as touch, smell and hearing, and how they can make you feel horny. They all play their role!

Foreplay involves anything that makes you feel sexy and horny. So that could start with creating the right bedroom environment, followed by lots of kissing and touching, wearing something sexy, and wrestling or teasing each other. Foreplay can have an influence on what might happen later, and so putting in some time at this 'starter' stage can make the 'main course' more appetising.

For centuries, people have used stimulants, legal and not, to enhance their sex lives or to serve as an aphrodisiac. All drugs, including alcohol, make you less inhibited and so more adventurous. But they could also encourage you to have riskier sex and be less likely to use a condom.[1] It is a personal choice, but if you do take drugs and have sex then be aware of the added risk and learn more about the drugs you take (see page 229).

It's pretty obvious when you are turned on because you'll start to get an erection. Plus you may feel your heart beating a bit faster and feel warmer. This is the body preparing itself for sex. Once you are turned on and hard, most guys can stay that way for 15 to 30 minutes – if the sexual tension is kept up too. It's usual that your levels of arousal will rise and fall during foreplay and your penis will do the same. How long you last depends on how aroused you are. Many men, especially when they start out, rush past foreplay and go straight for the guy's penis. This is a sure way of taking the action up a notch but you may have missed some fun along the way.

Exploring each other through talking, touching, kissing and simply enjoying the intimacy of a sexually charged atmosphere, can be as hot as the real action itself.

KISSING

'For me the kiss tells it all. If he can't kiss then unless he is very hot I'd find it really hard to get turned on enough to have sex. I can't imagine dating someone I couldn't have a good snog with!' Imran, 24

For some men, kissing is central to their sexual lives. Some even say that the kind of kisser you are predicts how hot you'll be in bed. Who's to say? But it's fun trying out. What is certain is that the lips and tongue are among the most sensitive parts of the body. Added to this is the fact that puckering up your lips and rubbing them against someone else's is a very intimate act, so it's not surprising that kissing is fully charged with emotion and meaning.

Some guys still find kissing an issue – even when they can enjoy all other types of sex without a problem. Some men just don't enjoy it. This can be a sign that they are not completely comfortable with their sexuality. For others, kissing may be reserved for their most important relationship and is not to be performed with others outside of that.

There are all types of kissing, from the quick, close-lipped peck to a full-on open-mouthed snog with tongues – called 'French' or 'deep' kissing. For most gay men all types of kissing just come naturally; it's hard to teach someone to kiss. It is normal to be nervous about kissing if you've not done it before – or even if you just feel that you're not as good as you'd like to be. But be reassured that practice does make perfect!

The basic rule is to try to relax, and to kiss someone as you would like to be kissed. Practically speaking, always go in at an angle or from the side. It can be more of a turn-on if you both keep your eyes open, or at least open them occasionally. If you like a soft kiss, gently brush his lips with yours. If you enjoy a deeper kiss, then once your lips meet keep your mouth open slightly and let your tongue explore and respond to his. Try also nibbling or gently sucking his tongue or lips. Like most aspects of sex, take it slowly – work up to the full-on tonsil tickler, don't just dive right in!

The uses of the basic kiss don't need to stop there. You can use it in all manner of other ways. Passing food or drink to one another – champagne or ice cream are favourites – can be a big turn-on during foreplay. Of course, you don't need to concentrate on kissing his lips alone – he has a whole body landscape to explore through kissing.

Love bites are a variation on the basic kiss. You do them by gently sucking up the skin between your lips or through gentle nibbling. Usually you do it around the neck. Some guys are very sensitive here and it can be a real turn-on, but these marks may be visible for several days and so may not be appreciated. You should never suck or nibble so hard that you draw blood!

Health risks

* Bugs that cause colds and flu are found in saliva and so can be passed on through kissing.
* Sexually transmitted infections (STIs), such as syphilis and herpes, can affect the mouth and be passed on by kissing. Avoid kissing (or oral sex) if you or your partner has any type of sore on the lips or in the mouth.
* It's probably not possible to pass other infections like gonorrhoea or chlamydia by kissing provided you don't kiss his penis or anus.
* HIV is present in saliva but current thinking is that the quantities are far too small to pose any risk through regular kissing.
* Bad breath – the medical name is halitosis – is never a turn-on. It's often caused by the bacteria that occur naturally on the surface of the tongue. Smoking, drinking and eating spicy foods all contribute. Paying attention to your oral hygiene is essential. It's important to keep your teeth clean, and flossing regularly and using an antiseptic mouthwash can also help to control the bacteria that cause bad breath. Snogging a smoker is usually an unpleasant experience so, if you smoke, have a pack of mints to hand!

PUBLIC KISSING

Gay men are now more able to show affection in public than they once were. Many give each other a kiss on both cheeks when they meet and some have no problems giving their boyfriend a snog on the street corner. But just as many gay men are shy about these displays of affection, or feel that they are too 'girly' for them. Unfortunately, in many parts of the country, kissing in public would prompt ridicule at the very least and could even be dangerous.

COMMUNICATION AND SEX TALK

'I went out with a really hot guy for a while and we had pretty good sex. But when fucking he just lay back and looked pretty bored and wanked himself off. I never told him but it started to annoy me and was a turn-off. I did try asking him how he was feeling and he would say he was enjoying it but I was never convinced! Maybe it was me but I've never had that experience before – or since. I like guys to show me whether I'm giving them pleasure and I do the same in return.' Dimitri, 28

Communication is essential to good sex – and should involve more than a final 'Have you cum yet?' Some men feel that they should naturally be able to guess what their partner likes and that asking a question is some kind of failure. But it's not. For others talking is a source of embarrassment as it makes them admit what they are enjoying and doing. You do not need to talk all the way through – that is likely to ruin the mood rather than heighten the arousal – but some communication during sex and about what you like and don't like will make things much better. Some men don't give any feedback at all during sex and that can make it seem stale and emotionless. So always give some response to what he's doing and say how much you're enjoying it. The same goes for what you're doing – tell him or show him your pleasure. If you can't tell whether he's enjoying something that you're doing then ask – but do it in a gentle and sexy way.

Communication doesn't have to be purely verbal. A moan or a groan when he's doing something you like can be just as good. Showing your partner what you like will encourage him to give you what you want. Try gently moving his hand to where you want it to be, or guide his lips and mouth. Sex can be noisy and some feel liberated by making loud primitive noises, whereas others hardly utter a sound. Neither way is right or wrong so try experimenting and see how you feel.

Some men love to 'talk sex' during foreplay and during sex itself. Describing what you are doing and what you're going to do can be a real turn-on for both him and you. Some go further and like the whole porn star thing – even the clichéd US accent – with lots of 'Oh yeah!' and 'That's hot!' Or you could tell your partner what to do, such as 'Suck that dick' and 'Fuck me/my arse'. But just because you go for this it doesn't mean that he will. It could be a complete turn-off for him. He may not see it as sexy but as funny or plain ridiculous. Be guided by his reaction. If it seems that he's not responding then stop or ask him if it's something he gets turned on by.

TOUCH AND MASSAGE

'I love it when he touches me – it is the way we always start out – and he knows it's what turns me on. The gentler it is the better.' Ashish, 27

Everyone knows the comfort of a good hug or a hand on the shoulder. Touch is an essential human action and has many meanings. At its simplest, it can make you feel loved and cared for. Just think about how you start any kind of sexual experience – it is likely to be with a touch. Once you have started, touching and being touched can often be the most emotional and intimate aspect of sex.

Touching is a way for you both to come closer together, to show affection and, during foreplay, to turn you on and get you aroused. The skin covering the human body contains thousands of nerve endings that sense touch in all its variations – a gentle stroke, a scratch, a tickle or a deeper rub, and not forgetting the pain and possible pleasure of a sharp slap. Remember that you can use more than your hands to touch – some guys use their feet, arms, whatever – so it's possible to touch someone with almost any part of your body.

Many men love to give or receive a massage and this is a great way to prolong and enjoy foreplay. It can also reduce tension and anxiety so that the sex that follows is more intimate and relaxed.

If you are into massage, pay attention to the practical aspects, such as the temperature of the room, and make sure you have the massage oil ready. You may want to put on some music or create a more erotic feel and play porn. Any part of the body can be massaged so it can get as horny as you want. Some parts of the body are more sensitive than others and during foreplay guys tend to concentrate on those areas. The inner thighs, genitals, nipples and anus/buttocks are the main areas but everyone is different. You'll soon find out which are his pleasure zones. The parts of the body that are more relaxing to massage are the head, back and shoulders. You don't need to use your hands alone but also your tongue, or lips, or devices such as dildos and vibrators (see page 127).

Different strokes provide different sensations, so when using your hands there are a few techniques that you might want to try. You can either straddle him to do these, or stand or kneel at the side.

Effleurage: These are long, smooth gliding strokes that you can make with the flat of your hand or the base of your thumb. Your strokes can go up and down the spine, for example, or from shoulder to fingertips. You can use this kind of stroke at the beginning of the massage, to spread the oil all over his body, and to really get to know his body and warm him up. Later you can apply a little more pressure *for a deeper* sensation.

Petrissage: This is more of a kneading, squeezing stroke, applying gentle pressure to work on specific muscles improving the flow of blood to the muscles.

Friction: This is the deepest kind of stroke – either circular or side-to-side – and made with the base of the thumb or fingertips. Do this the way you might rub your temples if you had a headache. It's a good stroke for working the muscles on either side of the spine to work out deep knots and tension. It is best done only once you have warmed up his muscles using the other strokes.

Tapotement: This is a sequence of sharp, rapid strokes and takes various forms. Hacking is done with the side of your hand, like delivering a karate chop. Beating uses the closed side of your fists, just as if you were beating a drum. Cupping involves using cupped hands and, with soft wrists, percussing rhythmically across his back. Slapping, when done rhythmically and softly, feels very good on large fleshy areas such as the backs of the legs.

Health benefits and risks

* As well as being intimate and sexy, massage usually enhances you sense of well-being. It not only relaxes the mind, but is also thought to improve blood flow to the muscles, reduce tension, aid lymph circulation and relieve muscular aches and strains. It's used for all sorts of medical problems, and to help alleviate stress and anxiety too.

* If you massage with your hands (and don't have any body-to-body contact) then the only slight risk is from a couple of minor STIs, such as syphilis, scabies, genital warts, herpes and molluscum (see page 143). These can be picked up and passed on through direct skin contact. If you keep your clothes on there's no way you will catch these. Otherwise touch and massage carry no risk of any other STIs.

* There are no risks of HIV transmission from the massage itself. However, if you are using body oils for massage purposes, take care to keep these oils well away from condoms if you plan to go on to have anal sex, as the oil will rot the rubber and may cause a tear. If you have massaged his penis, wash it with warm soapy water before putting a condom on. Silicone-based lubes are useful as they can be used for massage and don't harm condoms.

FROTTAGE

Foreplay usually involves a lot of rubbing, grinding and thrusting against one another – that's frottage. This can be so hot that you may cum while doing it.

There's loads of ways to enjoy frottage. You can lie front to front, or front to back, or rub up against any other part of his body. You can be clothed or unclothed or in any state in between!

Health risks

* Clothed frottage poses no risk to your health. Unclothed there can be a risk of passing on or picking up STIs that can be transmitted through direct skin contact.

* It can be easy to get carried away if you are naked and rubbing against each other. Then it's all too easy to start nudging your penis just inside his anus – or his in yours. HIV and other STIs can be passed on through pre-ejaculate (pre-cum) so keep your penis clear of his anus unless you are wearing a condom!

NIPPLE PLAY

The sensitivity of the nipples varies from one guy to the next. Some guys are wired up for pleasure and others are not. If your nipples are an erogenous zone for you then just having them touched, played with or sucked will be a treat. And some guys love to do the playing.

Men also vary in the different types of stimulation they like. Some prefer gentle strokes with a moistened finger. Try using lube or massage oil, which can increase the sensitivity of the nipple and often bring the most resistant one to erection. Other men like their nipples tweaked. Simply roll the nipple between your first finger and thumb, first clockwise and then anticlockwise. It can be enjoyable to have them nibbled or pulled too. As with everything else in sex, ask your sex partner what he likes, or try out different ways and see how he responds. You can also try more extreme forms of nipple play using clamps and weights (see page 130).

Many guys find that the more they play with their nipples – pulling or tugging them or using clamps – the more there is to play with. This can make them more enlarged as well as more sensitive to stimulation. Working on your nipples a few times a week may help. Or you could try a suction cup on your nipples to pull them out and give you more to work on. Some men find that having piercings makes their nipples more sensitive – and this often lasts even if you have the piercing jewellery taken out.

Health risks

* Nipple play is safe and poses no serious risk to your health, but never play so hard that you break the skin.
* Beware of coarse facial hair. The nipple is a delicate area and can chafe easily, which could lead to infection.

KEY POINTS

* Don't neglect foreplay! Spending time touching, kissing and exploring each other's bodies will heighten your sexual experience.
* Infections such as syphilis and herpes that can affect the mouth can also be picked up and passed on through kissing or oral sex.
* Frottage can pose a possible health risk if you have direct skin contact while naked as an STI, such as warts, molluscum or herpes, can be passed on.
* Communicating and feedback is essential to good sex. If you can't tell what's going well then how can you know that the right buttons are being pushed?

ELEVEN

GETTING IT ON

What constitutes 'gay sex' is really a matter of preference. For some guys it's anal sex, for others it could be a 'hand job'. In this section I'll describe the three most common sex acts that lead to orgasm – masturbation, and oral and anal sex.

MASTURBATION – ALONE OR TOGETHER

'I love to wank sitting on the end of my bed in front of a mirror but not able to see my face. I love to play with my nipples or rub my lower abs with my free hand, that feels really good.' Jean, 29

Many guys are brought up thinking that masturbation is wrong and dirty – a legacy of Victorian Britain where the church and the medical profession warned that it was a danger to the soul and even to your sanity! This guilt early on can affect how men feel about masturbating as adults – whether alone or with a partner.

Alone guys masturbate (or 'wank', 'beat their meat', 'jerk off' – you can choose your own terms) to relieve tension or sexual frustration, or just for the fun of it. There are so many ways, places and times that guys do it – just think about your own experiences for a start! Wanking to porn, watching yourself in a mirror, using a dildo – for many guys, wanking alone is an intimate and essential part of their sex lives where they can be selfish and focus purely on their own pleasure.

Masturbating with a partner is sometimes seen as a second-class sexual act compared to other types of sex. But wanking your partner off or wanking together can be very hot – if you allow it to be. You're probably an expert on how to do it to yourself and can cum easily. But it can be a little harder to satisfy a partner.

So how do you masturbate? The most common grip is to wrap your fingers around the shaft of the penis and work up and down, or you can reverse your grip so that your thumb is now on the underside. Or you could try using the other hand for a change of sensation. Simply rubbing the head of your cock into the well-lubed palm of your hand can also be very pleasurable, as can using a twisting action at the base of your penis – like opening a bottle of wine – and working up the shaft a little way.

There is another way, called the 'cock pull'. Start with one hand at the base of the penis and slide it up the shaft. Just as your hand slides off the end, you place your other hand at the base and slide it up to the top. Continue alternating like this, and try to get a good rhythm going. You can also do it in the other direction. There are literally dozens of other ways you can do it. In fact, there are websites devoted to the art of wanking!

When you are doing it for your partner you can stand, lie, or kneel next to him. Remember to use lots of lube. Try all the grips you can think of, vary the rhythm and watch his reaction. If he is not giving you much feedback, ask him how he likes it. Both of you might need to be a little patient because it is all too easy to give up on it if you don't get it right first time. Don't just focus on his cock. Some guys get a hit from a gentle tug on the balls or by slipping a finger inside the anus and massaging the prostate.

If you're masturbating together, wrap a hand around both cocks and take turns to work them. You can either sit facing each other or stand up – both ways work. Or you can wank each other separately. You can also try sex toys such as the double-headed dildo, which could add more of a spark if you're into that kind of thing.

Health risks

* Generally speaking, masturbating each other carries a very low risk of catching or transmitting most sexually transmitted infections (STIs) and no risk of HIV, so it's a perfect way to play.

✱ But never use someone else's pre-cum or cum to lubricate your own penis as it could get inside you urethra and pass on an STI, including HIV.

ORAL SEX

'I love the fact that I can give a great blow job – it's a real turn-on to know that no matter the guy, I am sure to get a smile on his face and see him writhing in pleasure from what I can do. I'm often asked how I do it – but I think it just comes down to practice, taking time and experimenting. Too many guys are nervous about getting it right and so rush.' Steve, 27

Also known as a 'blow job', 'giving head', 'going down', 'deep throat' or 'fellatio' – the fact that there are so many names for it just shows what a big part oral sex plays in guys' sex lives. There are also whole books devoted to the subject. Where and when to introduce oral sex into your sexual play is up to you. You and your partner don't even need to be fully undressed. This can add to the charge of the situation and makes it ideal for those times where there may be no possibility of more.

Some men don't need advice on how to give a blow job – it just comes from a natural instinct. But many feel they are lacking in technique or want to really master the art. There are good blow jobs and bad ones, as you might have experienced for yourself. One question that is often asked is how to suck a large penis without gagging.

The basic blow job: the vacuum method

Start by finding a position in which you have easy access to the whole of his penis and testicles – this could be standing or sitting, kneeling, or lying down by your partner's side, but experiment to find out what works best for you. Kneeling is a favourite and gives you control, but if you want to be more submissive he can straddle you while you lie on your back. Alternatively, you can lie top to tail – called 'soixante-neuf' or 'sixty-nine' – and work each other. You can compare techniques at the same time!

Don't just dive in. Build in some anticipation – play with his testicles or stroke his thighs. He'll get turned on by the fact that you are taking your time and it will give him a buzz just to know you are appreciating the look of his cock.

If he's not circumcised, gently pull back the foreskin – but take your time doing that too as the foreskin is very sensitive and fun to play with. Next, give a few licks to the head of his cock. Spend as long as you like there! Try licking the whole length of his shaft from base to tip, nice and slowly, just as you would a lollipop. Seek out the fraenulum – a very sensitive part of the head – and use your lips there, or tongue it gently.

Now slowly take him into your mouth and start to suck, but do it gently – you are not a vacuum pump. If you do it too hard it will be painful. Cover your teeth with your lips so that you don't cut the skin of his penis. Keeping your mouth in a tight ring, gently glide the head of his penis in and out of your mouth. The edge of the head, called the corona, is the most sensitive part, so concentrate on that. By keeping your mouth tight you'll also create some suction. Vary the rhythm and depth you take him in – try shallow and faster then deeper and slower. A steady rhythm is best if you want to bring him to orgasm. Don't be surprised if you get tired – it can be hard work so take a break if you need to! Most times you probably won't bring him to orgasm, but with practice you'll build up your stamina and be able to carry on long enough to bring him off.

Some men give very little feedback on how you are doing, so if it is not obvious whether or not he is enjoying it then ask him. He might say that it's 'too sensitive' or it's 'too good'. That can mean the sensation is too strong for him. Don't be offended as some men are just more sensitive in certain areas. Just change what you're doing slightly.

If he has a thick or very long penis, you'll probably only be able to take part of it in your mouth (unless you are getting into the advanced class, which will be covered later!). In that case it's best to keep one hand around the lower part of his penis and pump it to the same rhythm that you work the top of his cock with your mouth. A slight twisting motion with your hand feels good too. Remember that the head of the penis is the most sensitive part and so this shouldn't reduce his pleasure.

Tips for givers:

★ Remember that you have two hands so use them on other parts of his body. Work his nipples, stroke his thighs, or massage or slap his arse, or even use a finger or sex toy in his anus to stimulate his prostate. Many men like it if you gently wrap your index finger and thumb around the top of the testicles and gently pull them away from the body. Pulling the balls away from the body can also delay him coming. But not all men are into ball play, so again, be guided by his reaction.

★ If you're not keen on the taste of cock then try dipping it in honey, jam or something more glamorous, if it takes your fancy! Making his cock taste good will give you a natural incentive to give better head. Putting an ice cube or ice-cream in your mouth will give him a cold blow job that can really heighten sensation. But be careful not to get anything down his urethra, as this can cause inflammation and possibly a discharge a few days later. It's also best to avoid this if you are going to use a condom later on as you might use something that weakens the condom, unless you take care to wash his penis afterwards.

★ Breathe through your nose – you won't last long if you don't! A good technique is to breathe out as you go down his penis and breathe in as you go up. Or when you have his dick as deep as you can, open your mouth and suck air in as you move back up his penis to the tip. Then as you go down on him again, breathe out through a slightly opened mouth. This also cools his cock on the way up and warms it on the way down – and gives you a break from your usual vacuum method.

★ Humming while you suck makes a pleasurable sensation. Try it out. If you're the musical type, alter the pitch to vary the sensation.

★ Keep some eye contact now and then – letting him see you working on his dick can be a real turn-on. You'll also get a better idea what he likes most.

Tips for receivers:

★ Keep clean – an uncircumcised penis with smegma under the foreskin is a real turn-off for many. If you like your cock being sucked then always ensure you maintain good hygiene.

* Let him take control. There is nothing worse than a man who tries to ram his penis down the throat of someone who is not ready for it. You could make him choke and he might even bite down on you!

* Remember your partner's sexual needs – sucking on your penis may not be enough to keep him turned on! Show him that you're enjoying what he's doing – either tell him or make some kind of sound! And use your hands or mouth on him too.

* If he's not doing what you like, let him know. Telling him the way you like it will make him more willing to please you.

* He may not want you to cum in his mouth. Tell him when you are about to ejaculate and then pick up on his cues. If he moves his mouth away that means he's not into it.

Advanced class: deep throat

Deep Throat, released in 1972, was one of the most influential porn films ever made (but a straight one!). Featuring Linda Lovelace, it was all about a woman whose clitoris was found to be in her throat and so needed to take a penis deep into her throat to achieve orgasm. Hence this type of oral sex is now called 'deep throat'.

Many men love the idea of being able to take a whole cock inside their mouths, and just as many love to have their cock swallowed. But to master this technique takes some practice. What stands in your way is the gag reflex. This is a safety reflex that makes you heave when anything touches the back of your soft palate that isn't followed by you immediately swallowing. (You can find it by trying to make yourself gag!) It's there to stop any food or liquid going down your air pipe and to stop your breath going down your food pipe. As most dicks are longer than the distance from your mouth to your soft palate they are likely to make you gag when you try to take them down completely.

You can learn to overcome your gag reflex, however. Think of sword swallowers for a start! If the thought of deep throating is not high on your list of pleasures then you may not be able to relax, which will only make your gag reflex worse. Start slowly and be patient – it is not easy.

A key first stage is to get your position right. To avoid his penis hitting the top of your soft palate, where your gag reflex is strongest, you should direct his penis more towards the area of the throat that curves downwards. The best position for this is to lie back with your head over the side of a bed or table. This way his cock is angled more towards your food pipe and away from the back of your throat and soft palate. This helps the muscles at the back of your throat to relax. Kneeling over him facing towards his feet can work well, too. You need to have a patient partner – not one who just wants to ram it in without a thought. With time you may master the technique and then he'll be able to thrust his penis inside your throat for short periods of time.

Some men suck antiseptic mouth lozenges beforehand because they can contain a mild anaesthetic that numbs the gag reflex. Others say that drinking orange juice helps too. If you do deep throat, expect your throat to be sore for a day or two after.

Health risks

* Many gay men don't realise that you can catch almost any STI through oral sex: this includes chlamydia, herpes, gonorrhoea and syphilis. These infections can affect the throat and can easily get passed to the penis.

* It is now clear that HIV can be transmitted through oral sex, but only if an HIV-negative man performs oral sex on a man with HIV – probably not the other way round. However, the number of cases known to have contracted HIV this way is small and it is far less risky than anal intercourse without a condom. The virus is present in pre-ejaculate as well as semen itself and so can be absorbed if it gets inside your mouth. This is perhaps more likely if your gums are in an unhealthy state or you have cuts, sores or ulcers anywhere in or around your mouth. The risk of picking up HIV this way increases with the number of men you perform oral sex on, and whether you let them ejaculate in your mouth.

* Wearing a condom for oral sex will protect you. But this is not popular with many men. If you are HIV negative and want to 'give head' without a condom, don't let him ejaculate in your mouth and take his penis out if you taste pre-cum. Pay attention to your dental hygiene as there is a greater risk of HIV transmission if you have any ulcers or sores in your mouth or suffer gum disease. If you have HIV then don't ejaculate in your partner's mouth

RIMMING

By definition, oral sex also includes rimming (or anilingus) where you explore someone's anus with your tongue. For some it's a complete turn-on – both to do it or have it done – whereas for others it has the complete opposite effect.

If you're not into the smell or taste of an arse then it can make the experience nicer if he ensures he is clean. Gently washing the outside of the anus is a start, but many men also use a gentle douche to clean inside – at least as far as the tongue can reach!

Favoured positions to receive anilingus are to squat over your partner, or lie on your back with your knees pulled back to your chest. The area around the anus is very sensitive and so try gently licking around the area, letting your tongue go around and then inside the anus.

If you're into rimming but your partner isn't, it can sometimes cause problems. Talking about it helps. Try going slowly, for example by starting off close to but not actually on the anus, and getting used to that first. If it's the smell and taste that you don't like then make sure he's clean or use a food you fancy to make it tastier.

Health risks

* The skin around the anus is very sensitive and can be cut or grazed easily. When washing, avoid scrubbing yourself clean. If you feel your partner's teeth or beard chafing against you then ask him to stop.

* STIs can be picked up and passed on through rimming. Rimming someone with an infection, such as gonorrhoea, herpes, genital warts and hepatitis A and B, can mean you pick up the infection. If you're the one being rimmed then there is less risk to you – but you can still pick up herpes or genital warts this way.

* If you rim someone it's even easier to pick up the bacteria – such as salmonella and campylobacter – and parasites – such as giardia – that cause diarrhoeal illness and cramp-like abdominal pains. This is because these infections live in the bowels and pass out in faeces. No matter how clean your partner is, during anilingus tiny amounts of faeces will still be present around the anus and can be passed into your mouth. Luckily these infections usually

only cause mild symptoms. If they are more severe you may require antibiotic treatment.

* HIV is not known to be passed on this way. There is just a theoretical risk that there could be blood in the faeces or that you can bite him and so get blood in your mouth.

* Some men use a dental dam, or square of cling film, or place a square of latex cut from a condom over the anus to prevent them picking up and passing on any infection. However, this is not popular with many men because it cuts them off from the smell, taste and texture that they enjoy. It also reduces the sensation for the guy being rimmed.

DENTAL DAMS

Dental dams are a square of latex that is stretched across the anus forming a barrier to prevent any exchange of bodily fluids and so preventing the transmission of STIs. The squares of latex come in many colours and flavours and can be bought from sex shops or on-line. Some can come with adhesive to fix it in place leaving you 'hands free' to roam your partner's body.

Tips on using dental dams:

• Dams are not lubricated but you can use a bit of water-based lube on the anal side to help keep it in place and increase sensitivity.

• You can make your own dam from cutting a square of latex from a condom or using a square of cling film.

• Keep the dam in place the whole time and never turn it round as this then exposes you to each other's bodily fluids.

• Dental dams can be messy so keep tissue handy and dispose of it carefully.

ANAL SEX

'I've never been fucked – I did try it once but I don't think I even got his
cock inside before I had to jump off because of the pain. It's not for me,
no way.' Shaman, 24

Some guys only like to fuck and others only like to get fucked. Many prefer a bit of both. Some see being fucked as the ultimate gay sex act and liken it to losing their virginity. Most can remember their first time – either with pleasure or with regret.

Unfortunately, society sometimes portrays a negative image of the guy who enjoys being fucked and this is sometimes reflected in the words used. In this section I'll use top and bottom. But there are other words that are often used:

* Those who like to fuck: 'top', 'dominant', 'active', 'insertive' partner.
* Those who like to get fucked: 'bottom', 'passive', 'sub' or 'submissive', 'receptive' partner.
* Those who like to fuck and get fucked: 'versatile', 'both ways'.

If you are starting out you may be frightened of trying because you think it will hurt (which it won't, if done correctly) or are frightened by the possible health risks involved, such as HIV and other STIs. Anal sex, too, has always attracted the most homophobic hostility. Many gay men are called names that refer to anal sex as being wrong or dirty – think 'fudge packer', 'bottom bandit', or even milder, seemingly harmless remarks such as 'Backs against the walls, guys!' So it is common for some guys to want to get away from this image and shy away from the possible pleasure of anal sex. For others, anal sex is tied up with issues of power and dominance – the idea of being fucked means that they are no longer in control and are in some way inferior.

If you want to try anal sex, or tried it but didn't find it a pleasurable experience, here are a few tips on how to get started. Those who are experienced can jump over the first few sections to read what many men ask about – how to take a bigger cock and how to have better anal sex.

108

Why anal sex feels so good

Anal sex can bring two men together in a unique way. It can be both an emotion-ally and physically powerful act. Many describe being fucked as a very psychological experience; you have to relax and allow yourself to be dominated. But it is also a physical experience. The rectum is full of nerve fibres that can sense stretch. And close to the wall of the rectum is your prostate gland. It can be felt by inserting a finger a few inches into your anus, towards your belly button. This gland gets massaged by the action of anal sex and gives you a deep sense of pleasure. It's the male equivalent of the woman's G-spot. Guys on top get their pleasure from the friction on the penis inside the anus, and the thrusting brings them to orgasm.

Starting out on the road to anal sex

If you're interested in having anal sex, the best way to start is with some self-exploration. Knowing about your anus and rectum is really important in understanding what's happening when you're fucked. It may help to refer back to the earlier chapter on anatomy of the arse. The good thing about self-exploration is that you can go at your own pace and choose a time that's right for you. It will build your confidence and help you to understand your limits. You may feel that your arse is never going to widen enough for penetration but the anal canal can naturally stretch very easily – with time, patience and understanding.

With the aid of a mirror, take a look at your anus. Squatting while holding the mirror under you is a good way to see it. This may seem a bit embarrassing at first and you may feel that what you're doing is wrong or somehow perverted but it's not. It's your first step in really understanding how your body is built. Next, apply some lube to one of your fingers and explore the delicate ridges around the anal opening. This should feel pleasurable, because the area is supplied by thousands of nerve fibres.

Now, try gently inserting just the tip of your finger inside your anus. If that feels comfortable, try making circular movements with it just inside your hole. It's crucial to take your time. Breathe out as you push your finger in and try to stay relaxed. You can also try pushing down as if you were emptying your bowels. This can help to open up the external sphincter – the circular band of muscle that controls your bowel movements (see page 69). You may feel your finger coming up against a little resistance. This is your internal sphincter. Pause there. Give it time – it can take up to 30 seconds to relax completely. Once it does you should be able to gently push your finger in a little further. You may experience quite an intense sensation and may even get turned on. But not all men get an erection this way. If you do, masturbating while you explore your anus and indulge in a little fantasy can help you enjoy these new feelings.

If you're new to this, then that's probably enough for a first step. Gently take out your finger. If you have ejaculated, take a moment before you take your finger out. That's because the sphincter muscles naturally contract when you cum (you may have felt this when you had your orgasm) so give them a chance to relax again. You may feel that you want to defecate – this is a normal reflex. But it is likely to be a false sensation, caused by the fact that your rectum has been stretched a bit and so is telling your brain that it must be full of faeces when in fact it isn't. Just realising this can help you override this message with time. Each time you try, you'll feel more comfortable with the feelings and, importantly, more confident about what you're feeling.

Going further

If you're comfortable with how far you have gone up to now (for some this takes days, for others weeks) you might want to go a bit further and start inserting two fingers. Or you might want to explore with a dildo. The best type of dildo is one that's flexible so that it can negotiate the bends of your rectum. Just like the penis, dildos come in all shapes and sizes, so if you're just starting out then don't buy what you *want* to be able to take but something you know you probably *can*. When buying from a sex shop too many guys walk out with a size that's far too big – both out of ambition and out of embarrassment at not wanting to look like a beginner in front of the shop assistant. The plan is to get comfortable and work up the sizes to one that you are happy with. Don't start too far up the scale as you'll only have to go back to the shop to buy a smaller one (and you're unlikely to get an exchange!). Many guys prefer to buy dildos from on-line sex shops.

To be completely safe, you should go for one that is about the same size as your own penis or slightly smaller. You could try vegetables but these tend to be too hard (and cold) and don't necessarily come with the wide base that stops a dildo getting lost inside you if you lose your grip on it.

You'll probably have to find a new position for this. Any position where your legs are drawn up is good – such as squatting or lying on your side with your knees drawn up to your chest. This helps to straighten the natural curves of the rectum. Try to relax – this is meant to be fun, not a chore. It will be much more pleasurable, and easier, if you are turned on, so work yourself up a little beforehand.

Use plenty of lube! Gently press the dildo against the back rim of your anus and then slip only the tip inside. Just inside your anus you'll feel the dildo come up against resistance from the internal sphincter, just like before. As before, be patient and breathe. Pushing down with your pelvic floor muscles, as if you are emptying your bowels, can also help your external sphincter open more easily. Keep up a little pressure on the dildo and with time you'll feel your internal sphincter relax and the dildo will slip inside you. This may be slightly uncomfortable but should not in any way be painful. If it is, then stop.

You need to remember that your lower rectum isn't a straight tube. It starts straight but after just a few inches it soon curves towards your back. As previously described, this is because of the muscular rectal sling that bends your rectum. Squatting or lying on your side with your knees bent has helped to straighten your rectum. Now, after you have inserted the dildo a couple of inches, try to angle it more towards your back so that it goes round this curve. Take your time, breath and go slowly. If you feel any pain it means you are hitting the muscular sling, so stop, pull back a little, and adjust the angle.

If you feel comfortable with the dildo inside you, start to move it slowly in and out. As you get more comfortable and your confidence increases, go a little faster. You should feel a deep sense of pleasure as your prostate is stimulated. The sensations you experience might seem very strange. Many guys feel high and you may get turned on. If you want to masturbate do so – you will likely have a more intense orgasm.

Taking more

After a few attempts with a dildo you should feel more comfortable and understand the sensations. If you have been using a smaller dildo, you may want to progress to lifelike or bigger sizes. It's a good idea to increase the size only slightly – not make a huge jump. Take your time. It can take weeks or months for some guys to get comfortable with these sensations and the experience as a whole.

POPPERS (AMYL NITRITE) AND ANAL SEX

It is possible to use amyl nitrite, or 'poppers', when using dildos or having anal intercourse. This liquid, which can be bought in most sex shops, is sniffed out of a bottle (see page 244). Poppers relax the internal sphincter muscle, which you cannot relax voluntarily. This can be helpful but poppers do carry serious health risks. For example, when taken with other drugs, such as Viagra, they can lower your blood pressure to dangerously low levels. They can also interact with some medications used to treat HIV.

The real thing

You might be reading this because you're done with going solo, or you may simply want to get more out of anal sex. The first thing to think about is hygiene. For the ways to keep clean, see page 70. If it's your first time having anal sex with someone, you could start by straddling your partner or lying side by side, rather than going for other positions like lying on your back with your legs up, or lying on your front, which give you less control over what's happening. Apply a good amount of lube to the outside of the anus and your partner's penis. Although condoms are usually lubricated it's not enough for anal sex and good amounts of lubrication will make penetration much easier. Add more lube during sex as it gets absorbed and things can get dry again.

Gently lower yourself onto your partner's penis. Just as with the dildo, you'll feel some slight resistance from the internal sphincter just a few centimetres in, so stop and wait for the muscle to relax. You and your partner need a little patience here – often lacking at this time! Although your partner will want to get inside you and may be anxious about keeping hard, he has to go at your pace. You'll soon feel your sphincter relax and you'll be able to lower yourself gently down on his penis. Then, again just as with the dildo, be aware of the bend in your rectum. Squatting or being on your side with legs bent up should help to straighten the rectum slightly, but any discomfort you feel as he goes deeper means he is hitting this bend with his penis, so get him to come out a bit and then change your angle so that he aims it towards your back. Just go slow and his penis will gently nudge the bend out of the way until your rectum becomes straight.

Once your partner's inside you, move slowly up and down on his penis a couple of times. You should start to feel looser and more comfortable. With time, you'll be able to vary the pace and even move into a different position. You may surprise yourself with the noises and facial expressions you make. Being fucked can be both an intensely emotional and physical experience.

Finding the prostate

It's hard to find your own prostate but you can easily find someone else's. Get your guy to lie on his side with his legs drawn up, or on his back with his knees in to his chest. Insert a well-lubed finger into the anus a few centimetres and against the front wall you should feel a smooth rubbery swelling. Rub this gently, or tap it, and you'll soon know if you've hit the spot because it should give him a sense of pleasure. When you're being fucked you'll know when your partner is stimulating your prostate with his penis because you'll feel the pleasure it gives.

Tips for tops

It's not a matter of just sticking it in and hammering away:

Talk to him: You don't need to have much conversation, but asking him if he likes what you're doing is the first rule of good sex. Letting him know that you're enjoying his arse is also essential – you don't need to sound like you're in a porn movie but he'll get a rush from hearing the occasional comment. Remember that anal sex can be painful and you can even cause damage. So watch his face for an indication that he is not comfortable.

Work him up first: Fingering. Slowly insert one or more fingers into your partner – some guys really love this. It can also be a way to get him relaxed before fucking. Use well-lubed fingers or wear latex gloves and make sure your fingernails are neatly trimmed as they can easily scratch the anus. Try making slow, circular movements. You can give him added pleasure by massaging him over his prostate.

Rimming. You can warm up your guy by licking his anus or inserting your tongue into it. It's a hot act, and a real turn-on for some. But others are not into it and for them it's a real taboo. If you enjoy doing it or having it done then hygiene is important.

Getting him to feel confident that you're going to respect his hole makes it more likely that you'll have a good time. You'll also get a good idea how much he is into anal sex.

Use lube: The lining of the anus makes a small amount of anal mucus but not enough for fucking. By using lube you're less likely to cause any cuts or grazes. Water- or silicone-based lubes are best; oil-based ones can weaken condoms (see page 83).

Putting it in: If he's on his back, press on the back wall of his anus to get the head of your penis in. Once just inside you'll feel a slight resistance from the internal sphincter. It takes up to 30 seconds to relax – so watch his face or wait till he tells you it's okay to go further in. If you try to ram it past, his sphincter can go into spasm. This is very painful and will have him yelling at you to 'get out!' and you can even tear his anus, causing bleeding.

Going deeper: Once you're past the internal sphincter, remember that the rectum curves backwards because of the muscular rectal sling. Go slowly to gently straighten out his rectum as you penetrate deeper inside. Again, ramming into him is painful for him.

Hands off his cock! It's tempting, but don't work his cock as you penetrate him. If you do, his anal sphincter will tense and you will not be able to insert your penis. But you can kiss him and stroke the rest of his body.

Vary the rhythm: The first couple of thrusts should be gentle, to give the anal muscles a chance to fully relax, to straighten out the rectum, and to let your partner get used to the sensation. After that, vary the rhythm (don't just be a machine gun) and don't go in too deep. A lot of his pleasure comes from your stimulating his prostate gland, which is only a few centimetres inside. Going in further than that is unlikely to give him more pleasure. You'll just be knocking against another turn in his bowel. Try side-to-side movements to stimulate his prostate, or change your position.

Tips for bottoms

It's not a matter of lying face down with your butt in the air and just taking it…

Talk to him: Let him know what's going on in your body – what you like and what you don't like. Your face may not be saying what you're feeling, so give him some clues. Feedback for the top is really important. He wants to know that you're enjoying it and that you want more of it. This can only make things better. If you get any pain you should let him know so he can go easier or stop.

Taking it in: Breathe out when he inserts his penis and then focus on relaxing. Pushing down as if you're opening your bowels can also help to relax the anal sphincters. Give the internal sphincter time to relax – letting him ram straight in can tear it – and choose a position that allow the rectum to straighten naturally. You could also get him to angle his cock more towards your back as he goes in deeper to avoid the pain of him hitting that muscular sling that causes the bend in the rectum.

Hands off your cock! You might want to work it but don't. Wanking will make your anal sphincter tense – which is the last thing you need.

Positions for anal sex

Finding a position that suits you can make all the difference. If this is your first time as the bottom, you may prefer to opt for the straddle position because it gives you more control over what's going on. You don't need to stick to one position but can switch from one to another – for example changing from sex from behind to face-to-face sex. But there are lots of positions to choose from – here are just a few.

The straddle: He is lying down as you lower yourself onto his penis. You can keep more control and can take it as fast or as slow as you want. You also control how deep you take him. It's a good position if you're new to anal sex and a good start position to get the arse loosened up before going onto others.

The classic: This is also known as the missionary position. You lie on your back with your legs apart. Placing a pillow under your lower back can help to tilt you so that he has a better angle to enter you. He can control how hard and fast he pumps you. Of course you don't have to be on a bed but on a table, floor – you

TAKING BIGGER DICKS

Usually it's the width of a penis and not the length that's the problem. By using anal dilators or dildos of steadily increasing sizes you can work your way up to the size you want to take, but there could be a natural limit at some point and you may have to accept that your imagination is bigger than your anus!

Anal dilators are firm but slightly flexible penis-shaped sex toys, just like butt plugs or dildos, made from rubber or silicone. What is special is that they come in kits of increasing sizes. So you start with the smallest one and, with time, work your way up to the larger size – or to a size you feel comfortable with. They will allow you to stretch your anus so that you get used to the sensation and allow you to take larger objects or penises. They can be bought most easily on-line or you can use a dildo or butt plug that can also be bought on-line or from sex shops. Anal dilators are also prescribed by doctors for men with, for example, an anal fissure to help stretch the anus slowly without tearing.

name it. It's a good position to be able to see each other's expressions and you can kiss and touch each other as well. It is also a good position for stimulating the prostate.

Doggie style: Many like it from behind and there are lots of ways to be taken in this way. You can be standing, bending over a table or bath, on all fours, or lying on your front with a pillow to keep your arse up. The top can put his arm around you or hold onto your shoulders to get a deeper thrust. These positions tend to be more comfortable for the bottom and allow for a varied fuck from the top. He can keep his eyes on your butt – a big turn-on as he's pumping you, and add in a little spanking. The bottom can also move back and forth to do the pumping.

The spoon or side-saddle: Here you're both lying on your sides and you raise one leg to let him enter you. He can kiss you and masturbate you. It's a good position from which to get into doggie style.

The lift off: In this position, he's sitting and you lower yourself onto him. He then moves your arse up and down. If he's strong, you can go from here to a standing position. You can get support from a wall or the edge of a table. This is a good position to continue the kissing and so keep up the feeling of closeness.

Health risks

* All STIs can be caught from unprotected anal sex, including gonorrhoea, chlamydia, syphilis, anal warts, herpes and HIV (see page 143).
* Getting fucked (being a bottom) without a condom poses the biggest risk for catching HIV. It is the most common way for gay men to pick up the virus.
* Some men think that if they don't cum inside they won't pass on HIV. But the virus is present in pre-cum as well as cum. Using condoms for anal sex reduces your risk of catching all STIs, including HIV.
* Even if you already have HIV and have sex with someone who you know is HIV positive too, you should still use condoms to protect you against hepatitis and syphilis, which can be more serious and harder to treat if you have HIV.

Also, if you don't use condoms you may be re-infected with a different strain of the virus. This is called superinfection.

* A small amount of bleeding (seen as slight pinkish traces when you wipe your anus) is common after anal sex. This usually settles after a day or so.

* After anal sex you may notice blood on the outside of your faeces. This is usually caused by piles (see page 212). If you experience pain at the same time, it can indicate an anal fissure (see page 215).

FISTING

'My partner and I have been trying out fisting over the last few weeks. We started with big dildos but still haven't managed to get his hand in. And I've been really sore and had some bleeding the next day. I think I'm just too small for him because he hasn't got big hands!' James, 22

Fisting, as the word suggests, is where a whole hand (but could be any large object) is inserted inside the rectum and lower colon. Some men like to get fisted deeper than this but most are usually satisfied with the fist alone. It's a sexual act that you either fantasise about or shudder at the thought of. However, gay men who engage in fisting say that it's an intensely intimate and pleasurable experience. It's not without risk, but done correctly it can be a safe form of sex.

Most importantly, you need to do it with a partner who you can trust, and take your time. If you're not able to take large sex toys then don't try for a fist. You might want to use dildos or anal dilators and gradually increase the size. This can help by slowly stretching your arse so that, eventually, you'll be able to try to take his fist. But don't rush this and put your body at risk – it can take a while. Each time you try it only go to your limit – you always have time to try another day.

Most men prefer to wear latex gloves before inserting their fingers, but if you choose not to then make sure your nails are neat and tidy and take off any rings or other jewellery that may scratch the insides. Use lots of lube. Be aware that some lubes popular for fisting, such as Crisco, are oil based and so not safe to use with condoms. If you have been fisted then some of the lube will remain inside. If you then go on to have anal sex, it can weaken the condom. Silicone-based lubes and some water-based lubes that have been specifically designed for fisting are safe, but always double-check that the lube you are using is okay with condoms.

It is best to start off with a couple of fingers, or use sex toys of increasing size, to loosen you up. Always guide the finger or toy towards the tail bone to start with and then angle it forward. Then insert one finger, and then two, three and finally insert all four fingers up to the knuckles. Once he is comfortable, use a slow rotating motion that will gently stretch his anus further. If you want to insert the whole fist, slowly slide the hand in with the thumb placed against the palm. Once the whole hand is inside make a fist. At any time be ready to stop.

Once you have the whole fist inside, you can either decide to stop at that point or move the fist very gently in and out – but not all the way. Some guys like to have the fist go even deeper inside. This should be done very carefully by opening the fist and moving the hand in deeper, and then making the fist again. When you've decided that you've had enough, bring the hand out very slowly.

Health risks

* If you go on to have anal sex after fisting be careful about the lube you use. The oil-based lubes that are generally preferred for fisting will damage condoms so it is best to use a silicone-based lube instead.
* Many guys prefer to douche beforehand to clean out the colon. But take care as douching can irritate the lining of the rectum and colon (see page 70).
* It's normal for those who get fisted to have some mild pain or bleeding afterwards. The pain is usually due to a tear in your anal canal or the anal sphincter going into spasm after all that stretching. Taking a warm bath helps and you should heal within a few days. Avoid anal sex until you are back to normal.
* The main risk of HIV transmission is if there are cuts or sores on the fister's hand. This can result in infected blood being transferred to or from the fistee's anus. Wearing latex gloves will protect you both.
* If you experience sudden pain or notice bleeding while you're being fisted you should stop immediately and the hand should be slowly removed – no quick movement. This can be a sign that his hand has punctured the thin wall of

your bowel and is an emergency situation. Get to a hospital accident and emergency department immediately. The reason this happens is that about eight inches inside your body the bowel makes a sharp turn to the left. Whilst the penis can negotiate this bend, arms or toys may not and can tear the wall.

* For some guys, drinking or drugs are a part of fisting. But this is not to be advised. You need to be fully aware of how your body feels during fisting so that you can detect any problems immediately. Drink and drugs can numb any pain and make you less aware when something is going wrong.

* Finally, a lot of guys worry about anal incontinence – not being able to control the bowels – if they get fisted. It's true that using thick toys or being fisted can stretch the anal muscles. But they can stretch naturally to a large size and go back to normal again. It's only if you overstretch the muscles regularly and over a long period, or get recurrent fissures, that they can become permanently stretched and scarred, leaving you with difficulty controlling your bowels. This is rare, however, and regular pelvic floor exercises or Kegels (see page 65) can keep these muscles in shape.

KEY POINTS

* Masturbation carries a very low risk of contracting STIs and no risk of HIV. But never use someone else's pre-cum or cum to lubricate your own penis as it could get inside you urethra and you could contract an STI, including HIV, this way.

* Giving good oral sex ('blow job') comes naturally to some but others need practise.

* Tips for oral sex – go slowly, breathe through your nose, and hold the base of his penis to control how much of it enters your mouth.

* If you want to take in all the penis ('deep throat'), then position yourself so that his penis aims towards the part of the throat that curves downward and away from the top part.

* Most STIs can be caught through oral sex.

* If you are new to anal sex, start by experimenting alone, using your fingers or a dildo.

* Always give the anal sphincters time to relax or you risk damaging or tearing them. Be aware of what your body is telling you.
* Talk to your partner, and encourage him to talk to you.
* Use plenty of lube and always wear a condom.
* Experiment with different positions for anal sex until you find one that is comfortable.
* If there is any pain or bleeding during anal sex, stop immediately.

TWELVE

SEX EXPLORATION

Sex is a big world and gay men like to travel. Most find that as they get more confident with who they are and what they like doing their sex lives get better and better, and so it is natural to want to experiment.

In today's busy world, with all the stresses and strains that life brings, sex can become boring and routine if you keep to the same old tricks and habits. Varying what you do, when you have sex and who does what can keep it fresh. Trying out new ideas can help, too. Some of the practices described here might sound a bit extreme for you – but each one has a milder side. Some may not work for you but you can still have fun trying.

All the sex acts listed here can put your health at risk but these risks will be explained along with advice on how to minimise them so that you have the confidence to explore safely.

PORN

'I remember a guy at a club telling me that he and his boyfriend were going to have some sex photos taken. I thought it was a weird idea at the time, but now I'm having some shots done for my boyfriend.' Kieran, 30

Gay men are avid readers and buyers of porn. They like to use it alone and/or with their partners. With the growth of the Internet, there has never been more pornography available at the touch of a button.

At its most basic, porn is a useful way to get yourself sexually worked up and help you to achieve your orgasm. A lot of tension and sexual frustration can be relieved by reading/watching and masturbating using porn. It is also one of the most popular ways that many gay men explore their fantasy world and learn about what turns them on. This can help you to have a more fulfilling sex life because you'll become aware of your needs and desires.

Watching porn with someone can be a good way to start off a session of sex, to make sex more raunchy, or as a quick way to get you off. A disadvantage with watching porn with a partner is that once it is playing it may be hard to draw his eyes away from the scene – but on the plus side it is usually a good way to find out what turns him on.

Health risks

* Watching and buying porn can become addictive. If you find that you're spending too much time watching it, buying it, or searching for it on the Internet, then it is becoming a problem. Groups that help sex-addicted men can also help men reduce their use of porn (see page 263). Remember, using or creating porn is a way to heighten your sex life – not replace it.
* Some men reach the stage where they can't have sex without watching porn. Again, talking to a trained counsellor can help.
* It's possible to develop sexual hang-ups because you compare yourself or your performance to what you see in films. You start to think that that's the real world, and you don't measure up. So it's important to realise that porn is a fantasy world and not reality.

DIY PORN

'My partner and I like to take sexy pictures on our mobiles and then send them to each other for a "surprise" when we're at work.' Salvo, 30

Many men like to swap sexy pictures when they are cruising for sex over the Internet. With web cams, mobile phones and digital cameras this has never been easier! More and more gay men are being upfront about showing themselves in their full glory.

Many men also like to take porn-style photos of each other, or video their sex sessions. If you think you might like to try this, you may find it a bit embarrassing at first. But give it a little time and even the shyest man can get a kick out of taking or posing for a few shots or watching themselves having sex. This needs to be done with both parties' approval so decide beforehand what you are going to do with the film, files or tapes that you make as they could come back to haunt you a few years down the line!

Another popular choice is to have semi-professional sexy or harder-core photos taken – perhaps to keep for memory's sake for all that gym work you have put in, or as presents for boyfriends.

EXHIBITIONISM

'I love guys getting off by looking at me and worshipping my muscles – I'm well into getting watched when I'm doing it, too. It's just a thrill knowing that I'm turning them on. It's a bit of a power trip, I guess!' Adam, 28

Many gay men enjoy being looked at – that's why there are so many 'tops off' clubs and why gay beaches are crowded with guys who have spent the months at the gym beforehand getting into perfect shape. If you don't like to be looked at then I'm sure you like to do the looking. But exhibitionism is more than this. It's getting a sexual thrill out of being looked at.

Why exhibitionism is so enjoyable for some is hard to say, but it probably has something to do with breaking rules and taboos. Showing yourself off in a sexual way, perhaps especially when you're gay, is not thought of as 'proper' or 'correct' behaviour. So guys get a thrill out of breaking this 'rule'. Exhibitionism could also be linked with the rise of 'body culture'. Guys now spend so much time working on their image that they want to get attention as a pay-off for all their hard work. And with the explosion of Internet dating and sex sites, there have never been more opportunities to get your kit off and get a kick out of showing off to the whole world – often in the most revealing of ways.

Is this a turn-on for you? Why not try it? It can range from something as simple as taking your time undressing in front of your partner to doing a full strip act. If you've not done it before, you might feel embarrassed – it takes some degree of confidence. But you should get some feedback from him to show that he's enjoying what you're doing. If you're not into doing it yourself but want him to do it for you – just ask! That might be all he's been waiting for. Some guys love to be told what to do and how to show themselves.

Health risks

* None whatsoever – so enjoy! You're unlikely to get into trouble unless you start doing it in public! But if you send out sexual images of yourself, make sure they don't go to the wrong people.

TOYS

'I see going to a sex shop and having a look round as just the same as window-shopping for clothes around town! It's not embarrassing, and I get a positive feeling that I'm paying attention to my sexual life. But I've not made the mistake of trying to impress the guy behind the counter by buying something that has never been used!' Adrian, 28

Walk into any gay sex shop or browse on-line catalogues and you'll soon realise that, for many gay men, using sex toys is a big part of their sex lives. Toys can make sex fresh or just liven it up. Some guys feel that you shouldn't need a toy when you have the real thing. But toys don't have to be about replacing something you haven't got but about adding an extra bit of excitement.

Using toys is also a good way to explore your sexual feelings by yourself and build up your confidence. If you're new to activities such as anal or oral sex, using dildos and other sex toys can help you become more comfortable and confident. If you want to work up to taking a bigger cock or even a fist, then using dildos of increasing sizes can help you to prepare.

There is an ever-increasing variety of sex toys to choose from. But there are a few that have remained firm favourites. It is true that sex toys cost money, while sex is pretty much free – apart from condoms and lube. But spending some money on toys is likely to be a good investment. Most cost less than a few drinks and could well enhance your sexual life.

Simple handcuffs can add more to your sex life than you might imagine by helping you to play out lots of different fantasies. They are available in many different materials – some padded for comfort. Or you can use a scarf or belt, if you don't have the real thing. Make sure that whatever you use is not fastened too tight – you should always be able to get a finger inside the cuff. If you feel your hand starting to get cold or numb, remove the cuffs or fastenings straight away. In the case of cuffs, it always helps to have a spare key handy, just in case. While you may enjoy being cuffed, you must be able to trust your partner. Yes, you may fantasise about being fucked after a bit of a wrestle but your partner also needs to know that 'no' means 'no'.

Toys for your arse: dildos, vibrators, butt plugs and anal beads

A dildo is a motor-less sex toy, often shaped like a penis. You insert it into the anus. Dildos come in all shapes, sizes and colours imaginable, from small to life-size (such as a model of your favourite porn star's penis) to frighteningly sized. Manufactured ones are often made out of latex (rubber) or soft plastic and so are slightly flexible. They may be ribbed or textured, to increase the stimulation. You can also make your own or use whatever is to hand – carrots and aubergines are popular!

Vibrators are motorised dildos, usually battery operated. They vibrate – often at different speeds – hence the name. They can be penis-shaped but are also available in a range of shapes. Many are made of hard plastic or metal and so are firmer. Most dildos and some vibrators have a wide base that stops them from disappearing inside your anus if you lose your grip with lubed hands.

Double-headed dildos are about twice the length of regular dildos and have a head at both ends. They are designed so that two guys, arse to arse, can enjoy anal stimulation at the same time.

Butt plugs are a shorter and usually fatter version of a dildo. They always have a flared base to stop them getting lost inside your anus and tend to be more pointed. They are usually made of rubber or silicone, which is warmer and not so hard. Once inserted they are designed to massage your prostate as you move about and so give you a strong sexual sensation. It is a good idea to start with a small one and then try experimenting – they come in all sizes.

Anal beads, love eggs or Thai beads are strings of beads, usually made of rubber or silicone, and come in a variety of sizes. They can also be made of plastic, but these can have a sharp seam around them. Beads are gently placed inside the anus, and then pulled out one by one at the time of orgasm to heighten its intensity.

Health risks

* Anal mucus left on the outside of a sex toy can transmit sexually transmitted infections (STIs), including HIV, so never share toys during the same session. If you do plan to share toys, always cover with a fresh condom that is changed between each insertion. Afterwards, always wash them carefully in hot soapy water and then dry them completely.

* With double-headed dildos there is the risk that secretions may trickle from one end to the other while you are using them and so enter each other's anus.

* There is the risk that shop-bought or home-made sex toys, or bananas and carrots, can get lost inside the body. If this happens to you, don't panic! It will normally come out again if you squat down and try to open your bowels. Gently using a finger or two may also help. But be patient. However, if you experience any pain or if it doesn't come out after an hour or two, then go straight to the nearest hospital accident and emergency department. You may feel embarrassed but the staff have seen it all before – you won't be the first

and you won't be the last – so making up a story about 'slipping on the fruit bowl' is not worth it!

★ Home-made toys are more likely to break, or cut you, or cause an infection. So if you do make your own make sure it is clean, has no sharp edges, is not made of something breakable, such as glass, or won't give you splinters, such as wood.

★ Sex toys can damage the anal and rectal lining so use plenty of lube. Remember that oil-based lubes weaken condoms, so use silicone- or water-based ones if you plan to share toys or have anal sex after you have used the toy.

★ Forcing a sex toy is not only very painful but may also damage the anal sphincter and lining. Wait for the sphincter to relax first and angle it slightly towards your back to negotiate the curves in your rectal passage.

★ It is possible to puncture the wall of your bowel, especially with a large dildo, if you are being too rough, so if you experience any pain while using a dildo – stop!

★ It's quite common to see a little blood after using a dildo – especially if you have used a bigger size than normal. This will usually clear up after a day or so and is nothing to be concerned about unless it is heavy bleeding or doesn't stop. Other injuries are similar to those you can expect from anal intercourse (see page 117).

Toys for your dick, balls and nipples: cock rings, sounds, ball spreaders and nipple clamps

Cock rings are made of rubber, metal or leather and come in all sizes. They usually fit around the base of your penis and testicles, but some just fit around the penis. Blood enters the penis through arteries deep inside, but drains out via veins located close to the surface. Cock rings squeeze these veins shut, so keeping the blood inside, keeping you harder for longer and can also make the penis a bit bigger. With rings that fit around your testicles, always put your balls through first and then your penis. Many have adjustable straps that you secure around yourself.

Sounds are stainless steel wands – a little like knitting needles – that guys stick down the urethra. By moving them up and down they can bring themselves to orgasm.

Ball spreaders prevent the balls coming in close to your body and so stop you coming. This can both prolong and heighten your orgasm. They are made in a variety of materials including leather, denim and nylon.

Nipple clamps are shaped just like a regular clip. You attach them to one or both nipples and they can then be tweaked for stimulation. Clamps are better than a simple clothes peg because the degree of squeeze can be altered. Weights can also be attached to them for extra sensation or they can be made to vibrate by being attached to a small battery.

Health risks

* Cock rings need to be the right size. If it is too small it will cut off the blood supply to your penis and you may have problems getting it off. If it is too big it won't be tight enough to keep the blood in your dick. If you're new to this it's best to start with an adjustable one.

* A cock ring that you can't remove is a potential emergency. If you can't get it off, try putting cold water on your penis and testicles and using lots of lube. If you cannot remove it after an hour or so, or if you start to experience pain of any kind, seek medical attention.

* You can damage the soft tissues of your penis by wearing a cock ring for too long. Don't wear one for more than about 30 minutes and always take it off before you go to sleep.

* Inserting any object into your urethra can introduce an infection and there is the added risk that what you put in you won't get out. Never use a pencil or similar: you can easily tear the lining and this can lead to scarring that may make it hard to pee.

* Overuse of clamps can enlarge your nipples and give them a 'worked' look. It's also common to get a surge of pain once your nipple clamp is released. This is the blood rushing back in and feeding all the nerve fibres that have been numbed.

GROUP SEX

'Usually after clubbing there is always some "chill out", where a group of us get together. Some guys may start fooling around. At the first few I went to, I just sat around and chatted to my friends. Since then I've done some fooling around too – but it's not often that I really fancy all the guys. Usually I prefer to hook up with just one! But it can be good fun if you treat it as a laugh.' Marcus, 25

Many guys like group sex – or gang bangs – but probably even more men think or dream about it, or pretend they've had it! Threesomes are the most common. Either a couple will bring in a third guy to liven things up, or three men hook up together. But there can be, and often is, more than three.

Until 2003, sex with three or more men was illegal in the eyes of the law. Changes in the law have now made it legal if all men consent.

Being with lots of men can be a big turn-on. Some guys like to watch, or be watched. Some men like to do it with just one guy, and some like to mess with as many as they can get their hands on. When you have sex with more than one, it's usually just about sex and nothing else. So it's best to realise that from the start. If you've not tried it, you'll get a good idea of what can go on by watching porn. Most guys are nervous the first few times, so make sure it's something you want to do.

There are many combinations of what you can get up to – but here are a few:

Spitroast: Three men. One is fucked while giving a blow job to another.

Daisy chain: Any number of men from three upwards form a line where they are being fucked from behind and fucking the guy in front.

Double penetration: Being fucked by two dicks at the same time.

Isosceles lock: Three guys make a triangle to give each other blow jobs or wank each other off.

Health risks

* Having group sex – even without anal sex – obviously can expose you to extra risk of contracting STIs. Negotiating safer sex practices can also be more difficult when you're with more than one guy. Wear condoms – and use fresh ones for each partner.
* Drugs, which often play a role in some groups, plus the heightened sexual charge of group events, can lead to you taking greater risks than you would normally.
* You might feel under pressure to take part and do things you wouldn't normally do. Be sure that this is your kind of thing. Some men are into it and others aren't. Either just say it's not your thing and don't go along, or if you find yourself in a situation where it's heading that way, just leave. Never do something you don't want to do out of peer pressure. Respect your own choices.
* Feelings of guilt and jealousy often come to the surface after a group session. If you are bringing a third guy into your relationship, don't underestimate the effect this can have on you as a couple. Plan ahead and try to discuss why you want to do it and what you are both hoping and looking for. Many couples set ground rules about what kind of things they want to do, or agree on what to do if the guy you invite only likes one of you.
* And if you are the third one brought in, you may feel emotionally let down at the end as you leave the couple cuddling in bed. So you'll need to be quite strong psychologically.

FANTASY AND ROLE-PLAY

'We're into the Army look. I find it such a turn-on. It makes sex last longer and much more exciting. It might sound weird but we pretend to chat each other up like we've just met after some kind of training drill – it can make us laugh but it can be quite sexy, too.' Gary, 24

Your brain is your most important sexual organ. Lots of men fantasise when they're having sex, and not necessarily about the one they are having sex with. This is normal and natural.

You can use your imagination and explore your fantasies in the real world, too. You know how you feel when you're wearing something that makes you feel sexy, such as a particular pair of jeans, leathers, or swim trunks. Most gay men have an idea of what kind of guys they find hot – men in leather, military men, men in boots or suits, or in sports kit, white socks, or jockstraps. A man in Speedos is always a firm favourite! These images are often tied up with what is seen as very masculine. But it's not just the look, the smell and feel of them; some materials, such as leather and combat gear, are linked to our ideas of what is macho and manly.

Wearing a uniform often forms part of a fetish scene (see overleaf) but for many guys any kind of dressing up can be a big turn-on. Going a little further and actually playing a role can bring your fantasies to reality. You could really *be* that plumber coming to repair a dodgy boiler!

You may think that you haven't got a fantasy. Fantasies can take time to develop because, for some guys, they are buried under layers of inhibitions. Builders, policemen, bikers and hitchhikers … there are a lot to choose from.

You don't need to spend a fortune to get the right look – just use your imagination a little and improvise. If you're going to role-play, try to keep it as realistic as possible. If you start to giggle then any feeling of sexual arousal you have will soon disappear. Play it straight and you'll soon discover that fantasy and role-play can really work.

Health risks

* The beauty of fantasy and role-play is that, in itself, it poses no risk to your health so you can enjoy it without any worry. Just make sure that the sex you have is safe!

FETISH

'I go for guys in rubber – just the smell and look of it is a turn-on for me. I've been into it for ages but I've only just started going out on the scene, which is great! I didn't think so many guys were into the same thing as me.' Daniel, 24

A fetish is an object or form of behaviour that turns you on sexually but that is not normally regarded as being sexual. It goes beyond a fantasy for a type of clothing or going for a particular type of guy. It's more a sexual fascination or obsession. The fetish can be about anything really – army boots, socks, dirty underwear, or a particular part of the body, such as the ears or feet that they like to lick or have licked. Or it can be a type of behaviour, such as acting like an infant, or a smell, such as dirty jockstraps or armpits or leather.

Usually you'll know that you've got a fetish because you find yourself thinking about it all the time and masturbating to these thoughts and images. Why some people have them and others don't is hard to say. It may be that if an object or behaviour was linked to an early sexual experience it can stay connected. As an adult, you may want to re-enact that original experience and it becomes a source of great sexual pleasure or it may be that a non-sexual part of the body becomes a replacement for another part that is more normally seen as sexual. For example, the feet may become the focus of attention rather than the penis or nipple. Different parts of the body have their own special significance too. If your fetish is feet, you might like the idea of being dominated and being subservient because we use our feet to walk on or stamp on things.

Your sexuality should be fun, so it is important to let your fetish come out, just as long as it doesn't harm you or anyone else. If you don't, then it can become a burden. Talking about a fetish with a partner can be difficult but most guys have some kind of preference that others might see as slightly weird. With the growth of the Internet you will be able to find someone somewhere – and probably more than you think – who will share your fetish. If you can bring your fetish into your sexual life then it will provide a great source of pleasure.

Health risks

* It's common for guys to feel guilty, or even ashamed, about their fetish. But if it does not harm anyone else or put your own health at risk, then you should be free to enjoy it.

* The only danger to watch out for is that you start to focus on your fetish too much or that it starts to take over your life. Your fetish should not become so important to you that it starts to interfere with normal daily living or that you can't enjoy sex without it.

SADOMASOCHISM (S&M) AND BONDAGE

'I've slowly got into the S&M scene and now it's my main way of enjoying sex – well, it's not really sex as most guys would think sex is. But it is hard to explain what it's about! For me, it's about being in a sexually charged atmosphere and stretching out sex for a whole night.' Ryan, 35

Many men enjoy the odd slap, or fantasise about being tied up, or fucking or sucking off a guy that's been tied up. Men who are into S&M play get their sexual kicks from experimenting with behaviours involving domination and submission, role-play, stimulation and pleasurable pain. The kick comes from assuming these roles, often for hours, with more 'ordinary' sex acts taking a secondary role. Guys who are into S&M may also enjoy wearing certain clothing, such as leather, rubber, uniform, lycra, jockstraps or sportswear.

In S&M there is usually a dominant partner, known as the top, that enjoys being in control and giving out the orders. He will be the one who does the tying up, the spanking, and the cock, ball or nipple play. The submissive guy, the bottom, sub or slave, gets aroused by being dependent, vulnerable and controlled. Some guys stick to these roles during a session – but others enjoy being the top for some encounters and the bottom for others, often depending on who they are playing with or their mood at the time.

In the S&M world, encounters are often very thought out and planned well in advance. Sessions can last for hours or even days. S&M sessions, or scenes, can include a range of activities. In their mildest form they are the sort of activities that many guys will be familiar with and enjoy as part of their usual sex lives, such as wanking, sucking, rimming and fucking. They may also include more 'kinky' activities.

* Bondage: This focuses on restraint – from having just the hands bound to the whole body. In its simplest form, bondage is pretty common and can add a lot of spice to your sex life, for example, by using rope, or wrist and ankle restraints to tie your partner spread-eagled to the bed or keep them standing. Blindfolds and hoods can add to the feeling of helplessness and control. What follows is up to you. Often guys like to tease and wank off, or fuck the tied partner, but most S&M scenes tend to generate their own sexual momentum. This kind of play touches on the issues of dominance and submission that are central to the S&M scene.
* Cock and ball play is where guys get pleasure out of their penis and testicles being tickled, squeezed, stretched or struck. To go a step further, toys and gadgets such as ball spreaders are often used (see page 129).
* Some people find being spanked or flogged very erotic. Light strokes stimulate nerve endings, which can feel good. Harder strokes cause pain, which can result in the release of endorphins into the bloodstream, resulting in a natural 'high'. How far you take it is up to you.
* Arse play involves using fingers, dildos or butt plugs to stimulate the sensitive nerve endings in and around the anus.

Key S&M facts

Before deciding that you would like to experiment with S&M sex there are some key factors to consider:

* One thing I have learned from speaking to experienced S&M players is that S&M is not about abuse. It is an agreed consensual sexual activity that involves differing levels of erotic stimulation of the mind and body.
* Only play with someone you trust. If you are going to experiment with S&M, you must have absolute trust in the person you are playing with. So reserve

S&M play for a lover or one of your regular sexual partners, if you can. If not, ask your friends if they would recommend anyone.

★ Agree before the scene which activities you do and do not want to explore. There is a huge range of activities that can be classified under the broad range of S&M, and most of these have various degrees and levels of pain intensity. You need to decide in advance what you would like to try, and to what level, and discuss this with your partner. Potential activities include role-play, bondage, nipple-play, cock-and-ball-play, arse-play, spanking, flogging, hoods, blindfolds, gags, dripping candle wax on the skin, attaching clothes pegs – to mention just a few of the more common.

★ Agree to a special 'stop' word. It is absolutely vital that both parties have a clear signal that indicates that whatever is happening must end immediately. Just saying 'stop' or 'no more' might be taken as part of the role-play – so you need a special signal that tells your partner you really do want him to stop. There can be many reasons for using the stop word, such as feeling that you are being pushed beyond your limits, severe pain, pins and needles, cramp or numbness, breathing problems, anxiety or panic attack, because the scene is not what you thought it was going to be, or it is not enjoyable or making you horny.

★ Take things slowly. There is no rush, so take your time. Feel comfortable with what you are doing or having done to you. Take breaks out of the scene, if necessary. The more effort you take to make the scene good for both of you, the better it will be.

★ Discuss the scene afterwards. It is important to discuss how it went for you. You need to be honest with each other if you are going to develop scenes that are horny for you both.

Health risks

★ There is the risk of serious injury if you get carried away so care should be taken to avoid the major internal organs and structures, such as the stomach, kidneys, liver and spine. When hitting the body, you should generally aim for the large muscle groups of the back, chest, buttocks and thighs, and avoid hitting 'bony' parts, such as the joints, hands and feet – and never hit the spine or above the neck. Some reddening of the skin and a certain degree of pleasurable pain is quite common, even desirable, during a session. Often the skin is gently slapped at the beginning of the scene to stimulate the nerve endings. One of the aims of erotic stimulation is the release of endorphins to give a natural high.

* In S&M, it is possible to draw blood, which could lead to infection, including the transmission of HIV. If the skin is broken, deal with it immediately. Cleaning the wound and covering it with a plaster should suffice. Alternatively, find another part of the body to play with. At all costs you should avoid getting another person's blood, pre-cum or semen into the wound.

* Bondage can cause chafing or even restrict the blood supply. Never leave a bound partner on their own. Ensure that bondage materials are never too tight and check for pins and needles regularly. Never tie anything around the neck, as this could easily lead to accidental strangulation. Always be prepared to release bindings quickly if necessary. Keep a pair of bandage scissors to hand and ensure that you have spare keys for handcuffs and padlocks.

* Hoods, depending on their design, can restrict breathing. Never leave a hooded partner alone and always ensure that you can release the hood quickly, if necessary. Some guys get a big kick from using breath control, but this is dangerous and definitely only for experienced players.

* If you intend to share sex toys then use fresh condoms for each guy. A better idea is to have separate sex toys for each person.

* Mixing drugs and sex is dangerous. You may take more risks as your inhibitions and common sense melt away.

* You should be aware that in England and Wales it is illegal to engage in any sexual activity that causes injury, even if both parties consent. The current legal definition is that any marks on the body as the result of a sexual encounter must be 'trifling and transitory' for the encounter to be legal. General opinion is that this means marks lasting no longer than 20–30 minutes, but be aware these definitions have not been tested in the courts.

WATERSPORTS, GOB AND SCAT

'I went to a club the other week with a guy I met over the Internet. It was a Watersports club. I was pretty disgusted by what I saw but have to admit to being turned on.' Warren, 30

As part of your sex play, if you like to urinate on someone, or have them urinate on you, or you like to drink urine, you're into watersports. It's a type of fetish and some guys bunch it together with S&M acts. Gob is when men get sexual thrills out of spitting on each other and scat is when guys get a sexual thrill out of opening their bowels, or farting on a partner, or having it done to them. Some even go as far as eating faeces. It's often referred to as 'brown' in personal ads. A lot of guys find the idea of scat a major turn-off, so it can be a difficult subject to bring up.

Many guys do these sexual activities in the bath or shower. If you are going to do it in bed then a waterproof covering is advised! As with many of these sex acts, there are specialised clubs and groups who meet to practise what they like to do and these are easily found by searching the Internet.

Health risks

* Urine is usually sterile while in the bladder but it can pick up any infections that are inside the penis. HIV is thought to possibly be present in the urine, but not in sufficient quantities to pose a risk. However, to be safe, it's best not to get any urine on broken skin, or in your eyes or mouth.
* Don't urinate in someone's anus. Your penis should not be there without a condom on it anyway!
* Faeces can contain highly infectious bacteria, viruses and parasites, and so it is important to keep faeces away from cuts, sores, eyes and mouth.

KEY POINTS

* If you are into do-it-yourself porn, remember that you may not always have control over where the pictures, films or image files end up.

* Never share sex toys, unless covered with a condom, as this risks transferring STIs, including HIV.

* If you lose a home-made dildo inside you, help it to pass out by squatting and opening your bowels. If this doesn't work then go to your nearest hospital accident and emergency department.

* Don't leave cock rings on for more than half an hour or you risk damaging the soft tissues of your penis.

* Putting devices (called 'sounds') down your urethra can introduce infection.

* During group sex, remember to use fresh condoms for each partner.

* Bear in mind the effect that bringing in a third guy can have on an established relationship. Jealousy issues are just some of the problems that may occur, so discuss these possibilities with your partner in advance, and decide how you will handle them.

* Using your imagination through role-play and exploring possible fetishes can be a liberating and sexually rewarding experience.

* If you are into S&M play, do it only with those you can trust and avoid any activity that draws blood.

* Watersports, gob and scat can be safe provided you do not get urine, saliva or faeces into broken skin, mouth or eyes.

PART IV

SEX PROBLEMS

'I wish I'd known some of the things that can go wrong in sex when I first started! I've learnt by having a problem or two. I'd suggest that every guy tries to know a bit more than I did. It would have given me more confidence and stopped me panicking every time I thought something wasn't right – when, in fact, there was nothing to worry about.' Clifford, 28

When you're well and your body is working fine then it's easy to take your health for granted. But the slightest problem, especially when it has to do with your sexual organs, can send even the most relaxed and confident guy into a state of panic, fearing the worst.

It's fair to say that, like everything in life, sex is not without its risks or problems. Things can go wrong with your body, there's the possibility of picking up and passing on infections. Plus, as sex has so much to do with how you feel or think, your ability to enjoy it can be affected by emotional or psychological issues you might be dealing with.

This section is no substitute for getting medical care but will discuss the most common sex problems that gay men experience – from sexually transmitted infections to the problems of being a sex addict, and everything in between. Recognising when something is wrong or when things are just not working the way they used to is the most important – and often most difficult – step to take. Once you've made that first step it is usually clear what to do next.

Thankfully, when it comes to most problems related to sex, there are often good treatments and solutions available. Most men are embarrassed about talking about sexual problems, and many worry that any sex problem will immediately 'out' them to their doctor. This can discourage them from getting the help they need. But remember, you're not the first person with the problem and you won't be the last and many of the disorders described in this section are common to all men, no matter whether they are gay or straight.

THIRTEEN

SEXUALLY TRANSMITTED INFECTIONS

'I often get cold sores on my lips. A few months ago I had a similar type of rash around my arse, but it cleared up by itself. My doctor said it was probably herpes and that I need to think about telling my new boyfriend that I've had it. My doc says that I can still pass on herpes even when I don't have a rash.' Tom, 24

Sexually transmitted infections (STIs) are infections that you can pick up or pass on to others through sex. They can be caused by bacteria, viruses or parasites. Thankfully, there are treatments for all of them and most can be cured. Those that can't be cured, such as HIV, can now be controlled with drugs. Some STIs, such as hepatitis A and B, can be prevented by vaccination.

About 1 in 5 gay men (20 per cent) catches an STI every year.[1] Unfortunately, research shows that gay men are getting more STIs than before. Over 25 per cent more gay men are getting gonorrhoea now than they were a few years ago and over the last few years there have been many large outbreaks of syphilis –

a disease that had become very rare – in London, Brighton and Manchester.[2] With regards to HIV, the news is not good either. Over the last few years, the number of new HIV cases has been steadily rising. In the UK, men who have sex with other men (MSM) are still the group at greatest risk of catching the infection; this group acquired 3 in 4 (75 per cent) of all new cases of HIV in the UK in 2004.[3]

GETTING CHECKED

Many STIs don't have symptoms, so you may not know that you've caught one or that the guy you're with has one. Some STIs stay inside the body and do not show up till a long time after you were first infected. But if you feel that something is wrong you should get a medical examination. Many gay men have a full sexual health screening every six months, or annually, just to be sure. If you're having lots of sex it makes sense to see a doctor even more often. Research shows that about 1 in 2 gay guys (50 per cent) gets an annual check-up. Worryingly, though, 1 in 3 guys (33 per cent) has never had a check up at all.[4]

Never try to treat yourself! I have heard many horror stories about guys using detergent or lighters! Any embarrassment you may feel about having an STI will be far less than seeing a doctor after trying a 'home treatment'. And just hoping that things will get better by themselves is not a good idea either. Although the symptoms of the disease may go away, the infection itself may not. It can hide in the deep tissues and organs of the body, only to re-emerge and cause health problems later on. And in the meantime you will still be able to spread the infection to others. Finally having any STI also increases the chances that you will pick up and pass on HIV through unprotected sex. So getting treatment at the earliest opportunity is always the best option.

Where to go?
About 4 out of 5 guys (80 per cent) choose to go to a GUM (genito-urinary medicine) clinic, also called a GU or sexual health clinic, for tests,[5] and 1 in 10 (10 per cent) visits his own doctor. But GPs can often not provide all the tests you may

need, and if you have one STI it's possible that you may have another, so it makes sense to have a full check-up at a GUM clinic.

A GUM clinic can also offer vaccinations for hepatitis A and B, as well as HIV advice and testing, free condoms and lubricating gel, and support and information about all aspects of your sex life. The staff are well used to handling all kinds of sexual problem, so whatever your worry, don't hesitate to go. Some GUM clinics, especially in larger cities, have specific clinics for gay men, so you could book yourself into one of these.

Many men worry about keeping their visit to a GUM clinic confidential. Be reassured that all GUM records are confidential. They can't even be shown to your GP or insurance company without your permission. You can also ask to be anonymous, in which case you will be given a number.

You'll be able to find your nearest GUM clinic through directory enquires or through voluntary groups. You can also find it on the Internet (see Further Information, Resources, Websites and Organisations, page 263).

What happens during a visit?

Getting a check-up is easy. Once at the clinic you will usually see a doctor and/or nurse who will ask you questions about your sex life and about any worries you have. It can be embarrassing to talk about your sexual practices but it is important to be honest. Remember that everyone who works in a GUM clinic is well used to talking about sex. The next step is an examination. Don't be embarrassed when you're asked to drop your trousers. Again, remember that clinic staff have probably seen twenty other men that day.

Next, you will see a nurse for some tests. These can include swab specimens, taken from your throat, penis or rectum, a sample of your urine, and some blood drawn from a vein in your arm. Most clinics routinely offer an HIV test but this doesn't mean you *have* to have one. At all clinics, there are trained counsellors, called health advisers, to talk to you about the implications of taking the test and about what the result may mean.

Normally you will be given some results on the same day and may receive treatment. HIV tests usually take a week or two to come back from the laboratory. Some clinics can do HIV tests on the premises and you can wait for your result.

How you are informed about your result varies from clinic to clinic. Some clinics call you only if there is a positive result. Some send you a letter, and others ask you to come in person to receive your results.

What is the treatment?

The most common type of medication for STIs is antibiotics. It's vitally important to finish the whole course. If you don't, it's possible that not only will you remain infected but the organism responsible may develop resistance to the drug and may even become untreatable.

Also, do not have sex until you finish the treatment as you can still transmit the infection to others or become re-infected yourself.

You may need to go back to the clinic for further tests before you are given the all-clear.

Who do I tell?

Partners will need to be contacted so that they can receive treatment. This also ensures that they don't infect other men and that you don't get the infection back again. Depending on the infection, partners as far back as two years, sometimes even longer, may need to be contacted. But clinic staff will give you lots of advice on this. Having an STI can raise lot of problems that can seem worse than the infection itself. You may have to tell your boyfriend about a casual fling you had, or your infection may be a sign that he's been sleeping around. Telling others and making sense of it all can be difficult, but there are counsellors at most clinics who can help you sort through these issues.

Finding out that you have an STI doesn't necessarily mean that you or your partner has been unfaithful. For example, genital warts and herpes can stay in the body for years and may reappear at any time. Therefore the wart or blister you have today may be caused by an infection contracted years earlier and so is not a sign that you or he has been playing around.

Testing positive for HIV can be especially difficult to come to terms with. This is discussed on page 178.

GONORRHOEA

What is it?

Gonorrhoea (often called 'the clap') is a bacterial infection that can affect the mucous surfaces that line the penis, rectum, throat and even the eye.

How do I get it?

As the bacterium can be in your mouth, rectum or penis, you can catch it from all types of sex, but especially through unprotected anal and oral sex, and rimming. It's most easily passed from the penis to the throat or rectum. The bacteria is present in pre-ejaculate (pre-cum) and semen (cum).

How common is it?

Gonorrhoea is the second most common STI in gay men. In the UK in 2004 there were nearly 4,000 cases of gonorrhoea in men who had caught it from another man – a big increase compared with four years earlier.[6]

What are the symptoms?

Most men, but not all, get symptoms about two to three days after being in contact with the infection, but it can take up to ten days to see the first signs. The most common symptom is a green/milky discharge from the urethral opening at the end of your penis. Many men also experience a burning sensation when they urinate.

Other symptoms include sore throat, pain in the rectum, or pus coming from your rectum. Even the testicles can be painful if the bacterium spreads to them. In about 1 in 100 people (1 per cent) gonorrhoea spreads through the bloodstream to damage the joints, and in rare cases it can even cause heart problems.

How is it diagnosed?

Swabs will be used to take specimens of fluid from your throat, penis and rectum. These are examined under the microscope. The samples are also sent to the laboratory to be cultured (grown in a glass dish). There is now a test to detect gonorrhoea in a specimen of urine.

What is the treatment?

Gonorrhoea can be cured quickly and completely with antibiotics. Usually treatment is with a single dose of tablets or a single injection. The choice of drug usually depends on whether gonorrhoea was found in your anus, penis or throat. However, gonorrhoea is fast becoming resistant to standard antibiotics and so treatment also varies from area to area according to the particular strain of bacterium present in the region. Tests must first be carried out on the bacterium to determine the best antibiotic to destroy it.

Always finish the course of tablets and follow any other advice you may be given. Don't have sex until you are given the all-clear. Often you'll need to go back to the clinic a week or so later to make sure the infection has gone away.

If you ignore your symptoms, or fail to get treatment, or don't get the right treatment and fail to clear the bacterium, your symptoms may go away – but that doesn't mean the infection has. It can sometimes spread through your bloodstream to affect the prostate, and/or testicles, and in rare cases may attack your joints and internal organs. And you can still pass it on to others. So it's important to get checked and treated.

Who do I tell?

If you sought medical treatment because of symptoms such as a discharge from your penis or pain when urinating, then all your sexual partners over the previous two weeks will need to be contacted so that they can be checked. If you don't have any symptoms and the infection was only discovered during a routine sexual health screen, then all your partners over the previous three months will need to be checked. All sexual partners are treated, even if their tests are negative, because they are assumed to have caught the infection.

How do you prevent it?

Using condoms for anal and oral sex can prevent the spread of gonorrhoea. As it's possible to have gonorrhoea without knowing, regular health screening is a good idea.

NON-SPECIFIC URETHRITIS (NSU)

What is it?

NSU is any inflammation of your urethra (the tube that carries urine and semen out of the body). It's usually caused by the bacterium chlamydia (see page 151), which is the most common STI, but it can be caused by other organisms. Therefore, because the exact cause is not always known it's called 'non-specific'. Sometimes you may hear it called NGU or non-gonococcal urethritis, because the name is given to any cause of inflammation of the urethra except gonorrhoea.

How do I get it?

When NSU is caused by an STI you are most likely to catch it through having anal or oral sex without a condom.

However, NSU is not always sexually transmitted, so if your partner is diagnosed with this condition don't automatically assume that he has been playing around! Damage caused by having lots of sex or excessive masturbation can inflame the lining of your urethra and cause the symptoms of NSU, without there being an actual infection. Inflammation of your urethra can also be caused by a reaction to bubble baths or soaps – especially if you tend to scrub yourself clean. They can easily irritate and inflame the lining of your urethra, causing a discharge.

NSU can also be caused by non-sexually transmitted bacteria, as a result of putting an infected object down your urethra, for example, or having your penis pierced.

How common is it?

NSU is the most frequently diagnosed STI in gay men.

What are the symptoms?

Up to 1 in 2 men (50 per cent) with NSU has no symptoms and so does not know that he has the infection. If symptoms do occur, they usually appear about two to five weeks after initial sexual contact. The most common symptoms are burning pain when you urinate and sometimes a slight white discharge from the end of the penis.

Sometimes the infection can spread up your urethra into one or both testicles, making them swell and ache. Very rarely, the immune system can over-react to the infection, causing swelling and pain in your joints.

How is it diagnosed?

A swab is used to take a specimen from the end of the penis and this is checked under a microscope for signs of infection. This specimen is also sent to a laboratory so that the exact type and strain of bacterium can be identified. A urine sample may be taken as well, and tested to check for infection.

What is the treatment?

NSU is usually easily treated and cured with antibiotics. This can either be a single dose of antibiotics or a week's course, depending on which bacterium is the cause. Sometimes the antibiotic you are given may not work first time round and so you may need a second course.

As with other STIs, you shouldn't have sex while you're being treated or you can pass it on to someone else.

If you don't treat the infection, any symptoms will clear up, but that doesn't mean the bacterium has. Left untreated, or incorrectly treated, NSU may spread to your testicles or, rarely, cause swelling and pain in your joints.

Who do I tell?

If you had symptoms, then any sexual partners you've had in the last month need to be told so that they can be checked and treated. If you didn't have symptoms then, ideally, partners you've had in the last six months should be contacted. It's not easy telling partners about an infection. But you know it's the right thing to do. Partners are always treated, even if tests are negative, because they are assumed to have caught the infection.

How do I prevent it?

When NSU is sexually transmitted and so caused by a bacterium, always using condoms for anal and oral sex can prevent the transmission. But remember, NSU is not always sexually transmitted.

CHLAMYDIA

What is it?

This is a bacterial infection. It usually affects the urethra (the tube that carries urine and semen out of the body) but chlamydia can also affect your rectum or throat.

How do I get it?

Chlamydia can live in the urethra, rectum and throat so you pick it up or pass it on by anal and oral sex if you don't use a condom. Very rarely your eyes can be infected, too, if you touch them after getting the bacterium on your hands or if you get infected semen in your eye.

What are the symptoms?

About 1 in 2 men (50 per cent) get no symptoms at all – especially when the rectum or throat are affected – and so doesn't know he has the infection. If you do get symptoms, they will usually appear any time between two weeks and three months after sexual contact with an infected person. The most common symptom is a burning sensation when you urinate and you might notice a slight discharge from your urethra. Chlamydia can sometimes spread to one or both of your testicles, making them swollen and painful.

How is it diagnosed?

Usually a sample of your urine is checked for the infection but swabs are sometimes still used to take a specimen from your penis.

What is the treatment?

Chlamydia can be treated and cured with a course of antibiotics. As with other STIs, never have sex while you're still being treated or you may pass on the infection. If you don't get treatment, the symptoms may go but that doesn't mean the infection has. Chlamydia can spread to your testicles or rarely even your joints. And you can still pass on the infection to others.

Who do I tell?

If you have symptoms, sexual partners over the last month need to be told about your infection so that they can get tested and treated. If there were no symptoms and so you didn't know you had chlamydia (perhaps it was picked up during a routine sexual health screen) then partners from as far back as six months ago should be told. Partners are treated even if their tests are negative because they are assumed to have caught the infection.

How do I prevent it?

Using condoms for anal and oral sex can prevent the spread.

SYPHILIS

What is it?

Syphilis is a highly infectious bacterium that usually affects your penis but can also affect your rectum, or throat, or other parts of your body.

How do I get it?

The syphilis bacterium usually gets into the body through tiny breaks in the skin, especially around the anus, penis and mouth. So any direct contact with the sores or rash of syphilis can lead to transmission. Most often it is passed on through unprotected anal and oral sex, but also fingering, rimming, mutual masturbation or fisting can spread the disease if there is direct contact with the sores or rash. Recent studies show that almost 1 in 2 cases (50 per cent) of syphilis in gay men has been contracted through oral sex.

How common is it?

Syphilis has become much more common over the last few years with several outbreaks occurring in cities across the UK that have large gay communities. In 2004, there were over a thousand cases of syphilis in men who have sex with men (MSM), a massive increase from the 130 diagnosed in 2000.[7] Those most at risk are men who have lots of partners and who have sex in cruising areas or saunas.

How long does it take?

The first symptoms of syphilis can take from nine days to three months after contact with someone with the infection to show up – but it's usually around three weeks. But about 1 in 5 men never shows any signs of the early stages of syphilis.

What are the symptoms?

The symptoms of syphilis vary according to the stage of the disease. Syphilis has three distinct phases or stages.

During the first stage – called primary syphilis – you usually get a single sore or shallow ulcer (which doctors call a chancre) on your penis or testicles, or in your mouth or rectum. What makes this sore unusual is that it is usually painless and so may not be noticed – especially if it is inside your rectum. The lymph nodes ('glands') around your groin or neck may become swollen for a while. After a few days or weeks the sore will form a scab and then heal.

If you didn't notice you had a sore and/or didn't receive any treatment, within a few months you'll develop a red rash on your body, and especially on your hands and feet. This rash is *not* normally itchy. During this stage – called secondary syphilis – you may also feel tired and achy, as if you have the flu. You can also get mouth ulcers. Again, without treatment these symptoms clear up over a few months.

If you didn't receive treatment after the second stage, then once you recover you may not have any symptoms for a long while. But at any time from ten to twenty years later, you may go on to develop the third stage, called tertiary syphilis. In this stage your heart, brain and nervous system are seriously affected. If syphilis is acquired by a woman who subsequently becomes pregnant, the disease can spread to the foetus and the child may be born with serious physical disorders (congenital syphilis).

How is it diagnosed?

Thankfully, most cases of syphilis are now diagnosed during the primary or secondary stages. If a sore or ulcer is discovered, fluid is taken from it and examined under a microscope to identify the bacterium. If you have a rash, or any other symptoms that might be due to syphilis, then a blood sample can be taken to test for the infection. Testing for syphilis is also part of the routine sexual health screen that you get when you visit a GUM clinic.

What is the treatment?

The good news is that this infection can be treated and cured with antibiotics. But it usually requires a series of injections or a course of tablets over a few weeks to get the infection under control. Blood tests will be taken at regular intervals to check that you're responding to treatment. Once you've been treated, blood tests will always show that you've previously had the infection.

Syphilis is highly contagious and so you shouldn't have sex while you're being treated and until you've been given the all-clear.

Who do I tell?

If you are diagnosed with primary stage syphilis, sexual partners over the last three months need to be tested for the bacterium. If you are diagnosed with a later stage of syphilis, perhaps following the rash of secondary syphilis, or because it was discovered during a routine sexual health screen, then sexual partners from as far back as two years before will need to be tested. There is support and advice available at every GUM clinic about how to do this.

How do I prevent it?

Using condoms for anal and oral sex can help protect you from the most common ways of coming into contact with the sores of syphilis. But syphilis is highly contagious during the first two stages of the infection, and you should avoid even touching your own ulcer or rash to prevent it spreading to other areas of your body.

PUBIC LICE ('CRABS')

What are they?

Pubic lice are tiny crab-shaped parasites (hence the common name), about one millimetre long, that feed on your blood. The scientific name is *Phthirus pubis*. They usually live in your pubic hair at the base of your penis and around your testicles. But they can affect your underarm hair, and chest hair, or very rarely even your eyebrows or beard! The hair on your head is usually too dense for pubic lice so they can't survive there.

How do I get it?

Pubic lice can't jump or fly but must crawl from one infected person to another and so are almost always spread through intimate body contact, most commonly during sex. They don't survive long away from the body, so it's not really possible to catch them from sharing towels, or just sleeping in an infected person's bed.

What are the symptoms?

The main symptom is a severe itch, usually in the pubic region, which starts five days to three weeks after contact with an infected person. Sometimes you'll actually be able to see the lice crawling around. You might notice tiny black specks of lice faeces in your underwear, or the white specks of their eggs attached to your hair.

How is it diagnosed?

The severe itch is characteristic of infection with pubic lice, but seeing the lice themselves, or their faeces or eggs, will confirm the diagnosis. Sometimes confirmation is made by examining the louse under a microscope.

What is the treatment?

Some guys self-treat and shave themselves in the hope that this will clear the infection – but it doesn't work! To kill the lice you need a medicated lotion that you can buy from a chemist without prescription or get free from a GUM clinic. Popular ones are Lyclear or Derbac, but there are others.

You apply it to the whole body, avoiding the face and neck, and leave it on overnight before showering in the morning. The treatment should be repeated a week later to kill off any new lice that have hatched. If you have lice in your eyebrows you should seek medical advice. You should avoid close body contact while you're having the treatment. But washing clothing and bed linen is not necessary.

Who do I tell?

Current sexual partners need to be told so that they can get treatment, and all partners over the previous six weeks need to be warned to watch out for symptoms.

How do I prevent it?

It's very hard to protect yourself against catching pubic lice unless you have no intimate contact at all. You might notice a partner scratching his crotch or notice a rash, but this is unlikely! The best step is to check yourself regularly for signs of pubic lice and get medication if you notice any so that you don't pass it on to others.

SCABIES

What is it?

Scabies is caused by a pinhead-sized mite called *Sarcoptes scabiei* that burrows under your skin to lay its eggs.

How do I get it?

You need body contact to spread this parasite, so sex is a common way. But unlike pubic lice, it is possible to catch scabies just from holding hands or sleeping in the same bed as someone with the infection.

What are the symptoms?

The main symptom is a severe itch all over the body that's worse at night when you're warm in bed. The itch is caused by a mild allergic reaction to mite faeces, which gets absorbed into blood vessels, and not, as many people imagine, because you're covered in mites! Symptoms usually take two to six weeks to develop. But if you have had scabies before your symptoms may occur sooner – often just days after being in contact with an infected person. A rash usually develops a few days later, especially on the ankles, lower stomach or inner thighs. Lumps or blisters can develop around the genital area or even on your penis. Sometimes constant scratching of the rash can lead to infection.

How is it diagnosed?

Red lines or spots can be seen where the mite has burrowed under your skin. These are most often around your wrists or between your fingers, but any part of your body can be affected.

What is the treatment?

Scabies is easily treated with a lotion that you can buy from a chemist or get free at a GUM clinic. Popular ones include Lyclear and Derbac. You apply the lotion to your whole body – including the soles of your feet and hands, but not your face or neck. Leave the lotion on all night and wash it off the following morning. Repeat the treatment a week later. The itch from scabies can take a few weeks to disappear. That's because the mite has triggered an allergic reaction. A mild steroid cream such as hydrocortisone can help ease the itch. You should avoid close body contact while you're having the treatment.

Who do I tell?

Current sexual partners need to be contacted and treated and all the partners you have had over the previous weeks should be warned to watch out for symptoms.

How do I prevent it?

It's very hard to avoid catching scabies. Better to make sure you treat your own infection and that close contacts are also treated. It's not necessary to wash all your clothes or bed linen, although many people prefer to.

HEPATITIS A

What is it?

Hepatitis means inflammation of the liver. Hepatitis A is probably the least serious of the many hepatitis viruses that can cause this condition.

How do I get it?

This virus is very infectious. It is present in faeces and so can easily be passed to your mouth through sex acts such as fingering, rimming, handling sex toys or if you practise scat.

But hepatitis A is not only transmitted sexually. Most often it is caught by eating food prepared or handled by someone with the infection who has not washed his hands after visiting the lavatory. Abroad you can also catch it from water or food that is contaminated with faeces.

What are the symptoms?

Up to 1 in 2 men (50 per cent) with hepatitis A does not have symptoms. If symptoms do appear they start two to six weeks after contact with the infection. You may get a mild flu-like illness, and it can make you feel very tired. Some people become very ill and lose weight. You may notice your faeces are pale coloured and your urine dark. Your skin may feel itchy, and the whites of your eyes can turn yellowish (jaundice).

The illness usually lasts for one to three weeks and during this time your body will clear the virus naturally. Most people make a full recovery but for some it can take many weeks, sometimes months, before their energy levels are back to normal.

How is it diagnosed?

Hepatitis A is detected by a blood test. And at the same time other blood tests are carried out to check whether the virus is damaging your liver. A test for hepatitis can also tell whether you have had the infection in the past but have become immune to it.

What is the treatment?

There is no particular treatment for hepatitis A because usually your immune system deals with the infection. If the liver is damaged there are separate treatments for this. While you are unwell it is important to rest and drink plenty of fluids. Eat a low-fat diet and avoid alcohol, to rest your liver. Most drugs are broken down in the liver so it is best to avoid taking over-the-counter medication (including painkillers such as paracetamol) or recreational drugs. Up to 1 in 5 people (20 per cent) requires hospital treatment because of viral damage to the liver.

Unlike the other hepatitis viruses (see below), you can't become a carrier of hepatitis A, so once you've cleared the infection you can't pass it on to others. Also, once you've had the infection you are immune to it.

Who do I tell?

All your sexual partners during the two weeks before you got symptoms need to be told because it is during this time that you were most infectious and were passing the virus out in your faeces. Partners can be treated to prevent them getting the infection. If you did not get any symptoms and are found to have had the infection, say at a routine sexual health screen, then going back to the time when you think you may have picked up the infection is usually recommended.

How do I prevent it?

There is a vaccination against hepatitis A that can protect you. A single jab gives protection for about a year, or you can have a course of two injections six months apart that will protect you for ten years. Many people get the vaccination from their GP if they are planning to travel abroad to countries where the disease is endemic. So you can either go to your GP or visit a GUM clinic – although some clinics don't routinely offer it. A blood test may be carried out first to see if you have had the infection before and so are immune already.

If you have not been vaccinated you should avoid contact with faeces during sex. You can reduce your risk by washing your hands after handling condoms and sex toys, and using a latex barrier for rimming.

HEPATITIS B

What is it?

This is one of the many viruses that can cause hepatitis (inflammation of the liver).

How do I get it?

Hepatitis B is found in body fluids including blood, semen (cum) and pre-ejaculate (pre-cum) so it is spread when bodily fluids from an infected person enter the bloodstream of someone without the infection. Most often it is caught through unprotected anal and oral sex.

It is very infectious – up to 100 times easier to catch through sex than HIV. You can also catch it from sharing needles, razors, a toothbrush, and even cocaine straws or banknotes, because the virus can survive outside the body on tiny amounts of dried blood that can be left on these items and then pass into your bloodstream. The virus is also present in spit, so it may be possible to catch it through rimming and deep kissing.

What are the symptoms?

Most men don't have any symptoms when they get infected with the virus so they don't know they have it. If symptoms do appear they can start at any time from six weeks to six months after coming into contact with the infection. The symptoms are a flu-like illness including fever, general aches, nausea and vomiting and weight loss. You may notice your faeces are pale coloured, your urine dark, and the whites of your eyes may turn yellowish (jaundice).

For most sufferers, these symptoms usually pass after a few weeks as the immune system clears the virus from the body. But about 1 person in 10 (10 per cent) fails to clear the virus completely and it remains in the body. That person becomes a 'carrier' of the virus and so can still pass it to others. Up to 1 in 2 carriers (50 per cent) goes on to develop liver damage or liver cancer years later.

How is it diagnosed?

Hepatitis B can be detected by a blood test. The same test can also see if you are managing to clear the virus from your body, or that you've had the infection in the past and have become immune to it. Other blood tests are usually carried out to see how the virus is affecting your liver. If you become a carrier of the virus you will need regular blood tests and perhaps liver biopsies (where small samples of tissue are removed from the liver) to check for possible liver damage.

How is it treated?

Like hepatitis A, your body will usually clear the infection with time and so there is no special treatment given. Most people with the disease get through it by resting and avoiding anything that might cause additional damage to the liver, such as alcohol or recreational drugs. It can take a few months to get over the infection completely. But people who become very unwell need to be cared for in hospital. Fewer than 1 person in 100 (1 per cent) dies from hepatitis B infection at this stage.

If you become a carrier of the virus and tests show that it is damaging your liver, then antiviral drugs such as interferon and lamivudine are used. They do not cure the infection but can slow the virus down to allow the immune system to combat it. Rarely, the liver becomes so badly damaged that a liver transplant is necessary.

It can take up to six months for your body to clear the infection completely.

You should avoid sex until you are no longer infectious and have been given the all-clear by your doctor. If you become a carrier there are drugs that can help to control the virus and prevent your liver becoming damaged. In some cases, the body naturally clears the virus after a few years. But as a carrier you can still pass on the infection to others.

Who do I tell?

All your sexual partners in the six months before you got symptoms should be told, as they will need to be vaccinated against the virus. This can prevent them getting the infection or make their illness less severe. They may receive a series of injections of antibodies (immunoglobulins) that can stop them getting the infection. If you did not get any symptoms and your infection was picked up on a routine screen then it's usually advised to contact partners you've had from the time you may have picked up the infection.

How do I prevent it?

There is a vaccination against hepatitis B that can protect you. Gay men are at high risk of the infection so it's important to get vaccinated. The vaccine is free from any GUM clinic. You can also go to your GP, but you will then need to say why you need it.

Your blood will be checked first to see if you have already picked up the virus and become naturally immune. Otherwise you will need a course of injections, often over six months, although different schedules exist across the country.

Whatever your schedule, it's important to finish the course if you are to get fully protected. After the last injection your blood will be checked to see if you have a good level of immunity against the virus. Once you are immune you'll need a booster every five years or so to keep your levels of immunity topped up.

If you have not been vaccinated, using condoms for anal and oral sex can help protect you, and use a latex barrier when rimming.

Remember that you can't tell who has hepatitis B just by looking at them. Many people don't even know they have had the infection because it can be so mild. Even if they are carriers of the virus, they will often be completely healthy.

HEPATITIS C

What is it?
This is the most serious of the hepatitis viruses that can damage the liver. It used to be called 'non-A, non-B hepatitis'.

How do I get it?
Hepatitis C is present in the blood and so most often affects drug users who share needles and syringes. In the past, some people got it through blood transfusion. Blood is now screened for the virus and so there is no longer a risk of getting the disease this way.

You can also catch it through having anal sex without a condom, and through fisting or sharing sex toys. Men with HIV seem to pick up the virus more easily – but exactly why is not known.

It's also possible to contract the disease through sharing razors or tooth-brushes with someone who has the infection because tiny traces of blood may be left behind. There are even reports of people catching it from the tiny amounts of dried blood remaining on straws or banknotes used to snort cocaine.

What are the symptoms?
More than 4 out of 5 people (80 per cent) will not be aware that they have picked up the hepatitis C virus. If symptoms appear, they start any time from six weeks to six months after initial infection. There may be flu-like symptoms, and other symptoms, similar to those of hepatitis A and B. Only 1 in 5 people (20 per cent) clears the virus from the body naturally, so the majority become carriers. After many years, 1 in 5 carriers (20 per cent) will develop cirrhosis, or 'scarring' of the liver, or develop liver cancer.

How is it diagnosed?
Hepatitis C is detected by a blood test to look for antibodies the body has made against the virus. Once you have had the infection, these antibodies will always show in your blood. You may also need to have a liver biopsy (samples of liver tissue removed for examination) to see how much damage the virus has caused.

What is the treatment?

As with hepatitis A and B, no particular treatment is given for the initial symptoms of a hepatitis C infection. If you become a carrier, and tests show that it is damaging your liver, there are drugs that may slow the virus down and prevent further damage. Common drugs include interferon and ribavarin, but newer treatments are being developed all the time. You usually need injections three times a week for up to twelve months. However, fewer than 1 person in 2 (50 per cent) responds to these treatments. If you have hepatitis C you should limit alcohol consumption, or avoid it altogether, as it can increase your chances of developing liver damage.

Who do I tell?

If hepatitis C caused symptoms then all your sexual partners in the six months before your symptoms appeared need to be told so they can be tested. But as most people don't get symptoms, it is important to contact all partners you've had from the time you think you may have picked up the infection – many doctors recommend going back up to two years. If you become a carrier of the virus you'll always need to use condoms to prevent partners from catching the infection.

How do I prevent it?

Unlike hepatitis A and B, there is no vaccination against hepatitis C. Wearing a condom for anal sex and gloves for fisting will help protect you. Avoid sharing razors and toothbrushes, especially if you know someone has hepatitis C. The virus is especially dangerous if you have HIV. It makes the disease more aggressive and harder to treat, and can make HIV progress faster. If you inject drugs, never share equipment.

HERPES SIMPLEX VIRUS (HSV)

What is it?

This virus causes blisters, or ulcers, on the skin. There are two types of herpes virus: HSV 1 and HSV 2. It is type 2 that is normally regarded as a sexually transmitted disease because it causes blisters or ulcers anywhere around the penis (genital herpes) or in or around the anus (anal herpes). Typically, type 1 causes cold sores, which are blisters on the lips; however, it also causes up to 1 in 2 (50 per cent) of all cases of genital herpes.

How do I get it?

The herpes virus enters the body through tiny breaks in the skin. Almost all sex acts cause a bit of skin damage and so you are at risk of getting the virus if you have any direct contact with the herpes blister, for example, through kissing, oral and anal sex without a condom, rimming or fingering.

Once inside the skin, the virus travels down the nerves to the nerve root where it stays. It can reactivate at any time and travel back up the nerve to cause symptoms at the same point where it entered the body. If your partner has developed symptoms of herpes for the first time it doesn't necessarily mean that he has been unfaithful. He might have caught the infection a long time ago but has only now developed symptoms.

The virus can be shed from the skin of anyone who has the infection, even if they do not have the tell-tale blisters. In fact, up to 1 in 2 herpes cases (50 per cent) is caught from direct skin contact with someone who does not have an active blister but who has had herpes in the past.

How common is it?

It is thought that up to 1 person in 5 (20 per cent) has the genital herpes virus in the skin, but most don't develop blisters.

What are the symptoms?

It usually takes two weeks to develop symptoms after you have been in contact with a herpes blister. But it is possible not to develop symptoms until many years after the contact. Tingling or redness in the affected area is a first warning sign of the infection. A few days later, a crop of small blisters containing clear fluid usually appears on the skin. These burst and turn into shallow sores that are usually very painful to touch – especially the first time it happens. Over a couple of weeks they dry out, scab over and heal. Herpes can also cause flu-like symptoms, backache, headache and swollen lymph nodes ('glands') in the groin.

Sometimes you may only notice one or two blisters and they may not be very painful so you may not realise you have herpes. Many people just feel a little uncomfortable or have what looks like a small graze or cut on their skin.

After healing, the virus remains in the body but lies dormant in the nerves. That means you can get another attack – or a recurrence – in the same place at any time. Many people learn to recognise the warning signs of the infection. They often feel a tingling in their skin a few days before the blisters appear. Recurrences aren't usually as bad as the first time, don't last as long, and usually become less frequent over time.

How is it diagnosed?

A swab is used to take a sample of fluid from your blisters. This may confirm the diagnosis but it can take a couple of weeks to get the results. Therefore the diagnosis and decisions about treatment are usually made on the appearance of the typical blisters that herpes causes.

What is the treatment?

There is no cure for herpes but there are drugs that can help to ease the symptoms. The most common one is aciclovir, taken as a tablet five times a day for five days. Ideally, you need to start this treatment as soon as you see the rash or it will not help you.

The blisters of herpes can be very painful. Many people find sitting in a shallow bath of salty water helps, or rubbing petroleum jelly (Vaseline) or placing an ice pack wrapped in a tea towel on the blisters. Wearing loose-fitting cotton clothes and taking painkillers can also ease the discomfort. Another common remedy is placing cooled tea bags on the blisters.

Rarely, the virus can spread to the brain, causing meningitis (inflammation of the lining of your brain). This requires emergency hospital care. Typical symptoms of meningitis are fever, headache, neck stiffness and finding light painful.

Who do I tell?

You should tell all current and previous sexual partners, if possible. You should avoid having sex until your blisters have healed completely, as that is when you are most likely to pass on the infection to someone else. But even after the blisters have gone you are still infectious because the virus can still be shed from the skin.

How do I prevent it?

Unless the man you're with has an obvious blister it's impossible to know whether he has herpes and he can still be shedding the virus from his skin. Using condoms for sex can help to protect you, but the blisters of herpes can appear anywhere on the groin area or around the anus, and condoms do not cover the entire area.

If you or your partner has active blisters then avoid coming into contact with them, or better still, don't have sex of any kind until the blisters are completely healed. This includes cold sores around the mouth, so avoid oral sex or you risk spreading the cold sore virus to the genitals.

Herpes sores go away but the virus remains in the body. It just goes dormant in the nerves. Subsequent episodes are not usually as bad as the first, and knowing how to deal with it helps. If you get frequent attacks then there are tablets you can take that may reduce the chances of recurrence. These are similar to the ones used to treat a first episode, but contain a lower dosage. Factors that can trigger reactivation include illness with another infection, friction against the skin, for example, skin-to-skin contact during sex, or from clothing, or ultraviolet light through sunlight or sun beds.

GENITAL WARTS

What are they?

Genital warts are growths on the skin caused by the human papilloma virus. You can get them anywhere in the genital region, most often on the head or shaft of your penis, as well as around your anus or inside your rectum.

How do you get it?

The virus is transmitted by direct skin contact with a wart on another person. That can happen during most types of sex. Just rubbing up against a wart during foreplay can transmit the virus. But it is not very infectious and so if you are in contact with a wart it doesn't mean for sure you will go on to get one. It is also possible to pick up the virus from someone even when there are no warts visible because the skin continues to shed the virus from time to time.

How common is it?

It's thought that more than half the population probably has the wart virus in their skin but many don't develop warts.

What are the symptoms?

If you have been in direct contact with a wart, it can take between one and nine months for a wart to appear on you. But warts can develop even many years after the contact. The wart starts off as a tiny pinkish fleshy lump that, over time, can grow into a larger cauliflower-like growth. You can have one or a crop of them. It is usually painless but may itch. A wart inside the anus can bleed when you open your bowels.

How is it diagnosed?

A genital wart has a very characteristic appearance and so doctors and nurses can tell by just looking. If there is any doubt then a small part of the wart can be removed and examined under the microscope.

What is the treatment?

Treatment depends on where your wart is located and what it looks like. Your doctor will decide which is the most suitable treatment. If your wart does not cause any symptoms or bother you in any way then there is no need to treat it – but many people want them treated because they just don't like the look of them. Most treatments will take a few weeks to work.

The following are the most common treatments:

Creams: Podophyllotoxin (known as Warticon) and podophyllin get rid of the wart itself, and imiquimod (known as Aldara) may clear the virus from your body. You can get these creams free from a GUM clinic or on prescription from your GP.

167

Cryotherapy: This involves freezing the wart with liquid nitrogen and is an effective treatment. It involves a few trips to the GUM clinic. Cryotherapy is most often used when the wart is inside the anus.

Surgery/ laser therapy: In some cases, the wart is surgically removed or burned away using laser therapy, just like an unwanted tattoo (see page 47).

Although the wart will disappear after treatment, the virus that causes it can persist in the skin for several years, and so the wart may return at any time. This varies from person to person. Overall warts return in 2 out of 5 cases (40 per cent). Unfortunately there are no tests to tell whether your wart will come back after it has been treated.

See your doctor sooner rather than later. Like all STIs, warts are easier to treat at the earliest possible stage. Don't try to treat warts yourself. Guys have been known to cut them off or try to burn them. Don't! You'll only make the problem worse.

Who do I tell?

While you have a wart it is important to avoid spreading the virus, so avoid any direct contact. However, by the time it appears it is likely that you have already passed the virus to your partner. With casual partners, using condoms may reduce the chances of your transmitting the wart virus.

How do I prevent it?

Avoiding direct skin contact with genital warts and wearing condoms if the warts are on the penis and/or inside the anus may help to prevent you picking up/passing on the virus. But remember, as many guys have the virus in their skin but don't have warts.

MOLLUSCUM CONTAGIOSIUM

What is it?

This is a skin disease featuring pearly-white bumps or lesions known as papules. It is caused by a virus called a poxvirus and can affect any part of the skin.

How do I get it?

You can pick up the molluscum virus simply from skin-to-skin contact. This can happen during sex but you can also catch the virus just by touching the papules, and from contaminated clothing and towels. It is very common among children and is easily spread in changing rooms, swimming pools and saunas.

What are the symptoms?

Molluscum appears as painless firm, pink, waxy bumps about the size of a match head. These often have a slight dent in the centre. It can take anything from a few weeks to a few months for molluscum to develop after contact with an infected person. The bumps can occur anywhere on the body but when caught during sex they tend to be found at the top of the thighs or around the anus and lower stomach. Typically, you'll get a crop of less than twenty molluscum bumps and they tend to occur in clusters.

How is it diagnosed?

Molluscum bumps have a very characteristic appearance and so health professionals will be able to recognise them easily just by looking.

What is the treatment?

Molluscum will disappear without any treatment within a year of getting it because your immune system is able to fight the virus. Usually the bumps heal completely but occasionally they'll leave a small scar or lighter patch on the skin. Many guys don't like waiting that long. You can try gently squeezing them as this forces out the central plug. But this plug will contain lots of virus particles and is highly infectious so be careful not to get it in contact with other parts of your skin or you will spread the disease. Wash your hands thoroughly afterwards.

If you visit a GUM clinic the bumps can be removed by freezing (cryotherapy) or destroyed by piercing with the tip of a cocktail stick dipped in iodine or phenol. However these treatments are more likely to leave small scars.

How do I prevent it?

Avoid skin contact with the lumps or sharing towels with someone who has molluscum. If you already have molluscum don't scratch or fiddle with the lumps, or shave the area, as this will spread the virus.

BOWEL INFECTION

What is it?

This is any infection of the large intestine, or bowel, caused by bacteria such as a shigella, campylobacter or salmonella, or by parasites such as giardia, amoeba or threadworms.

How do I get it?

The infectious organisms are found in the faeces. During sex it is possible to get tiny amounts of faeces in your mouth, or on your hands and then pass it to your mouth. This is most likely during rimming or fingering, or through sex toys, or if you practise scat (see page 139).

What are the symptoms?

A bacterial or amoebic bowel infection produces typical food poisoning symptoms: stomach cramps, vomiting, fever and smelly diarrhoea, sometimes containing blood. Giardia causes bloating and very smelly farts. Threadworms can cause itching in and around the anus, particularly at night, and you may see the worms in your faeces, which look like tiny white threads of cotton. How quickly the symptoms occur depends on the particular bug, but can be from 24–36 hours to several days after infection.

How is it diagnosed?

The symptoms will suggest the most likely diagnosis. But to be sure of the exact organism a sample of your faeces will be sent to the laboratory to be tested.

What is the treatment?

In many cases the only treatment required for infections caused by bacteria, giardia or amoeba is to drink small amounts of clear fluid and take over-the-counter painkillers. Most cases clear by themselves within a few days. If your symptoms are serious or you have a fever then it's best to see your doctor as soon as possible so that a sample of your faeces can be tested to see which bug is responsible. If your symptoms don't clear up naturally then antibiotics or antimicrobials can be used. Threadworms are treated with an anthelmintic drug, such as mebendazole or piperazine.

How do I prevent it?

Avoiding contact with faeces is the most important way to avoid getting an infection. You may choose to use a dental dam or a square cut from a condom for rimming, and wear latex gloves for finger play. Simple measures such as washing you hands and keeping sex toys really clean can also help to reduce the chances of transferring the infection to your mouth.

Who do I tell?

Current partners need to be treated for their own sake and because you risk catching the infection again from them.

LYMPHOGRANULOMA VENEREUM (LGV)

What is it?

LGV is an STI caused by a type of chlamydia bacterium.

How do I get it?

Most cases of LGV are from unprotected anal sex but you can also catch it from oral sex.

How common is it?

It is more common in parts of Africa, Asia and South America. But over the last few years it has started to spread into Europe. The first case in the UK was in 2004.

Up to the end of September 2005 there had been a total of 215 cases of LGV.

Most of these cases were in London and 4 out of 5 guys (80 per cent) with the infection also had HIV.[8]

What are the symptoms?

The symptoms vary according to the stage of the infection. There are three stages:

Stage one: This starts between three and thirty days after sexual contact with someone with the infection. During this stage, a painless shallow blister or sore may appear where you came into contact with the bacterium. The usual places are on the head of your penis, and in your mouth or rectum. In some people this sore does not appear or they don't notice it when it does.

Stage two: The second stage starts one to four weeks later as the bacterium begins to spread. The lymph nodes ('glands') around your groin become enlarged and tender and you may feel feverish, achy and generally unwell. If your rectum is infected then you can get a discharge from the anus, bloody diarrhoea, and it may be painful to pass faeces. If your penis is affected then you may see a discharge from your urethra.

Stage three: If you don't get treatment by the second stage, the infection can progress to a third stage in which the disease spreads to the rest of the body.

How is it diagnosed?

LGV is still very rare and so it is generally only considered once other possible causes of the symptoms, such as syphilis and herpes, have been ruled out. Swabs are used to take specimens from the infected sites for laboratory examination.

What is the treatment?

LGV can be treated with a three-week course of antibiotics. But for full recovery the disease needs to be diagnosed before it has reached the third stage. As with other STIs, you shouldn't have sex while you are being treated or you will pass on the infection.

Who do I tell?

All current and recent sexual partners should be contacted so that they can be treated as well.

How do I prevent it?

Using condoms for anal and oral sex can protect you against the infection.

HUMAN IMMUNODEFICIENCY VIRUS (HIV)

What is it?

HIV attacks the cells of your immune system, called CD4 cells, so that you gradually lose the ability to defend yourself against certain types of cancer and infections. The infections are called 'opportunistic' infections because the organisms that cause them don't usually cause disease in healthy people but do so when HIV has damaged the immune system. When this happens you have what's called AIDS, which stands for acquired immunodeficiency syndrome.

HIV is an extremely serious disease that claims many lives each year. However, it is not the bad news it used to be. There are powerful drugs that can slow down the virus and help prevent the transition to AIDS. These drugs can help you live a normal life.

How do I get it?

The HIV virus is present in bodily fluids, especially in semen (cum), pre-ejaculate (pre-cum) and blood, and so is spread when some of these fluids get from a person with HIV into the bloodstream of someone without the virus. Most gay men catch HIV from unprotected anal sex. The chances of you catching the virus are greater if you are penetrated by someone who has HIV, especially if he ejaculates inside you, rather than if he is penetrated by you. This is because the lining of the anus is very thin and easily torn, causing bleeding, and also because it can absorb infected semen even if it is not damaged.

It is now clear that you can also catch HIV from oral sex. Your risk of catching it is much greater if someone infected with HIV ejaculates in your mouth, but the risk is still lower than from unprotected anal sex.

You can also catch HIV from sharing needles and drug injecting equipment because of trace amounts of blood left on the needles.

How common is it?

By the end of 2004, nearly 34,000 men in the UK diagnosed with HIV caught it from having sex with another man. Of these, 13,000 have progressed to AIDS and nearly 10,000 have died.

What is even more worrying is that the total number of new cases of HIV in the UK every year is going up. In 2000 there were about 1,507 new cases and in 2004 there were 2,185 new cases diagnosed. That is a 45 per cent increase in the number of gay men getting infected in just four years. Many of the new cases are in towns and cities with a large gay men community, such as London, Brighton and Manchester. Some research shows that up to 1 in 10 gay men (10 per cent) in London is HIV positive. What is perhaps more alarming is that up to 1 in 3 gay men (33 per cent) doesn't know he is positive.[9]

What are the symptoms?

In many people, the first symptom is a flu-like illness that appears from two to four weeks after they have been infected with HIV. This is called 'seroconversion illness' because it happens at the time that the body starts to make antibodies to the virus. Typically, these early symptoms of the infection are a sore throat, fever, headache, muscle aches and diarrhoea. However it is very easy to miss these symptoms because they are similar to flu and other viral infections. Some men have no early symptoms at all.

It can then take many years before more serious symptoms appear because initially the immune system is able to mount an effective attack against the virus, although it can't clear it completely. Over time the virus starts to wear down the immune system, and especially the CD4 cells, until it reaches the point where you can't fight off other infections and so start to become ill.

ARE YOU EXPOSED TO HIV?

If you think that you have been exposed to HIV, for example, if you have recently had unprotected sex with an infected person, there is a treatment that might destroy the virus before it can take hold. This is called post-exposure prophylaxis (PEP).

PEP is a month's course of two to three HIV drugs that you take every day. They can have side-effects and 1 in 4 people (25 per cent) suffers side-effects such as nausea, vomiting and diarrhoea. The treatment can stop you being permanently infected with the virus, although it doesn't work in every case.

To get PEP you must visit a GUM clinic or hospital accident and emergency department within 72 hours of possible exposure, but the sooner the better. You'll need to speak to a doctor to see if treatment is possible in your case. Be warned that the treatment may not be available in all parts of the UK. If you leave it later than 72 hours it may be too late, as the virus will have multiplied and spread too far inside the body.

The fact that PEP is now available should not make you think you no longer need to practise safer sex, but it can help those who have genuine condom accidents.

How is it diagnosed?

HIV is usually diagnosed by means of a blood test but there are newer tests that can detect the virus in saliva or urine. The blood test works by detecting antibodies to the virus, not the virus itself. If antibodies are found in your blood you are said to be 'HIV positive'. This means you have HIV and can pass it on to other people. If you don't have HIV you are said to be 'HIV negative'.

It can take up to three months for these antibodies to show up in your bloodstream. This is called the 'window period'. If you have a blood test during this time it may give a false negative result. It is not until the three months is up, when your

WHY SHOULD I HAVE AN HIV TEST?

More guys are getting tested for HIV than ever before – which means that more are being diagnosed early on in their infection. However, research shows that up to 43 per cent of gay men have never had an HIV test.[10]

Having a test is a big decision and one that only you can make. It's important to think through how you would cope if you had a positive result. However, there are good reasons why you should be tested sooner rather than later.

To begin with, if you do test positive you can start treatment at an early stage, which can help protect your immune system. Many people don't need treatment straight away but their health can be monitored closely so that they receive medication as soon as they need it. Also important, you can take special care to avoid spreading the virus to other people, and can inform sexual partners of your HIV status.

Where do I get a test? There are three places where you can have an HIV test. Most men go to a GUM clinic and there are some specialist clinics for gay men. Other guys go to their GP or to a private clinic. GUM clinics often have trained counsellors on hand who can talk through all the issues, and all tests carried out there are completely confidential – your GP won't be told the result unless you say so. If the test is done through your GP, the result may be put on your files and could cause problems if you apply for a mortgage or life assurance. However, your GP is not able to disclose this information without your saying it is okay to do so.

The HIV test result usually takes a week to come back but in some places it is possible to get the result within an hour. This is called 'point-of-care testing'. A tiny drop of blood is taken from the end of your finger and put on a testing strip. The strip will tell you whether you are positive or negative in about 15 minutes. The Terrence Higgins Trust is one of the organisations now offering these tests. For details, log on to their website (see Further Information, Resources, Websites and Organisations, page 263).

body will have had time to make antibodies against the virus, if present, that you can rely on the accuracy of the test result.

What is the treatment?

There is no cure for HIV infection – and many gay men have died from AIDS. But HIV is not the automatic death sentence it used to be. There are good treatments, called antiretroviral drugs, that can reduce the amount of virus in your body and so slow down the damage it does to your immune system. Many guys taking these drugs are now living long and healthy lives.

Treating HIV is complicated. Usually you begin drug therapy only once the virus has started to damage your immune system. You'll probably need to carry on taking drugs for the rest of your life. However, the virus can become resistant to the drugs you take. This is more common if guys don't take their drugs at the right time or miss doses. Sticking to antiretroviral therapy is not easy. Some drugs have unpleasant side-effects (although rarely serious) and some drugs have to be taken at different times of the day, either with, before or after food. However, sticking to your drugs schedule, and so keeping the virus under control, is getting easier. Many new drug regimes involve fewer pills and only need to be taken once a day.

STIs and HIV

Having HIV can affect the way that STIs (and other diseases) behave.

Syphilis: If you have HIV and pick up syphilis you are more likely to get multiple sores. The treatment you will receive may be different and perhaps last longer but you can still be cured of this infection.[11]

Hepatitis C: If you have HIV then it is more likely that you will pick up hepatitis C and you are more likely to suffer liver damage and at an earlier stage. Also, the treatments for eradicating the hepatitis C virus are less effective.

LGV: Most cases of LGV in Europe so far have been in guys with HIV. The reason for this is not fully understood.

Herpes: If you have HIV you are more likely to have ulcers that last longer. The treatments are usually just as effective, although you may need a longer course.

Warts: The virus that causes genital/anal warts stays in the body longer and can sometimes be harder to treat if you are HIV positive. It is also thought that having the wart virus makes it more likely to develop cancer of the anus. But this is still rare.

Molluscum: Guys with advanced HIV can get molluscum on their faces, whereas usually the disease only affects the body.

Who do I tell?

When you have an HIV test you will be asked to think about who you can rely on for support if you have a positive result. It is important to think through how you would react no matter how low you think the risk of you having the infection is.

Getting a positive test can be a huge shock for some. Other guys are not surprised. There is plenty of professional help available. Most clinics have advisers that can help you deal with the result and the impact it can have on your personal and work life. Telling others can be especially hard. Some decide never to disclose their status but this can limit the support you have.

Telling others

Most clinics will have trained advisers to talk to to help you decide who you may need to tell – including past or current sexual partners. Telling past, current or future sexual partners about being HIV positive is never easy – though some may argue you're obligated to do it – but thinking and talking through the issues can help you to make an informed decision that you feel comfortable with.

How do I prevent it?

HIV is not as infectious as many other STIs and is not automatically passed on or picked up. It's important to know that no-one is known to have caught HIV from sweat, urine or faeces. Although HIV has been found in these substances there is not thought to be enough of the virus to enable it to be passed on to others. The chances of you picking up and passing on the virus depend on factors such as the kind of sex you have and how long for.

Receptive anal sex

Receptive anal sex (being fucked by someone who is HIV positive without a condom) is the most risky type of sex. Semen (cum) and pre-ejaculate (pre-cum) contain the HIV virus and the lining of your anus is designed to absorb fluids and so can easily absorb the virus straight into your bloodstream.

Many men want to know the exact chance of acquiring the virus this way. Some research shows that if an HIV negative man has receptive anal sex with an HIV positive man then there is a 1 in 30 risk that he will pick up the virus.[12] But there are many factors that can affect this risk, such as how long the sex lasted for, whether it was rough sex or not, or how infectious the man with HIV was. These figures don't mean that you can have unprotected sex twenty-nine times and use a condom on the thirtieth and you'll be safe. You could be infected the very first time you have sex without a condom.

It is important to realise that you do not need to damage the anus in any way for the virus to be absorbed, but if you have anal intercourse for a long time, or you have rough sex so that your anal lining is damaged, this greatly increases your risk. This is because if you have damaged the lining it is easier for the virus to get into the bloodstream.

Some guys think that just inserting the penis for a short time or not ejaculating inside the anus makes it safe. Pre-ejaculate contains the HIV virus and so just 'dipping' in and out will still put you at risk. Using condoms for anal sex will reduce your risk because they provide a barrier between you and your partner.

Insertive anal sex

Insertive anal sex (fucking a guy who is HIV positive without a condom) is the next most risky type of sexual behaviour. Tiny amounts of blood in the rectum from anal sex and mucus secreted by the anus can contain the HIV virus and enter the other partner's body through the lining of the foreskin or the mucous membrane that lines the inside of the urethra. Any activity that causes more bleeding inside the anus increases the risk of getting HIV, such as not enough lube, having sex for a long time, the presence of anal warts, or cock-piercing jewellery. Using condoms for anal sex will reduce the risk because they provide a barrier between you and your partner.

There is also some research that shows that uncircumcised men are more likely to catch HIV than circumcised men when having unprotected sex. This is probably because the inside of the foreskin can absorb the virus more easily. But circumcised men get HIV too, so it is always important to use condoms.

Sex toys and fisting

Sharing sex toys and fisting also carry a big risk of contracting HIV. If a guy with HIV uses a dildo there may be anal mucus and blood on the surface. If you use this dildo yourself without washing it thoroughly or using a condom you are putting yourself at risk of catching HIV and other STIs.

If a guy has fisted a man with HIV and then fists another man without first washing his hands or changing his gloves, traces of blood and mucus will be transmitted from one man to the next. Again, if you damage the lining of your anus using toys or fisting it becomes even easier for the virus to enter the body. Never share a sex toy, or if you do share, use a new condom for each partner or wash the toy thoroughly between partners. Wear gloves for fisting and change gloves between partners.

Oral sex

It is now known that it is possible to pick up and pass on HIV from receptive oral sex (sucking the penis of someone who has HIV). It's not clear how many men have caught HIV this way but the numbers are likely to be very small compared to anal sex. There are dos and don't you can follow to reduce the risk of getting HIV from oral sex.

If you don't have HIV:

* Do practise good dental hygiene to keep your mouth healthy as HIV is more likely to be transmitted if you have mouth ulcers or sores, or gum disease.
* Ideally use a condom for oral sex. The more often you perform oral sex the greater your chance of getting the virus this way.
* Don't brush your teeth or use mouthwash just before you perform oral sex on someone.
* Don't let your partner ejaculate in your mouth as the virus may enter through cuts, sores or the mucous lining of your mouth and throat. Stomach (gastric) acid will destroy any virus that passes into the stomach, so it makes little difference if you swallow or spit.

If you have HIV:

* Ideally use condoms for oral sex.
* Don't ejaculate in your partner's mouth.
* Don't receive oral sex if you have any cuts or sores on your penis.

Other sexual activities

So far, there are no known cases of HIV being passed through water sports. All other forms of sexual contact, such as kissing, body-to-body contact, massage and mutual masturbation, also carry no risk of HIV transmission.

INJECTING DRUGS AND SHARING NEEDLES

HIV is present in blood, so if you share needles you are providing a very effective way of transmitting the virus. Tiny amounts of blood are left in the syringe that will go directly into your bloodstream. If you do use drugs, never share needles. Clean needles are available from needle exchanges and so there is no reason to share.

The future of prevention

World-wide, the HIV epidemic is costing millions of lives and millions more are infected or getting infected with the virus. Research into a vaccine against the virus is ongoing but is proving elusive. Most scientists now believe one will become available, but not for many years, and when one is ready it is unlikely to offer total protection.

Another way of trying to prevent the spread may be through microbicides. These are gels or creams that can be inserted into the rectum before sex to try to prevent transmission. There is one for use in the vagina currently being tested that may be available in about five years, but is unlikely to offer complete protection. It may stop transmission in some cases and could also be used with condoms to reduce the risk from condom failure.

KEY POINTS

* Surveys show that about 1 in 5 guys picks up an STI every year. Thankfully most STIs can be cured.

* In gay men, rates of STI, especially syphilis and HIV, are continuing to rise.

* Many STIs don't cause symptoms and so regular health screening is a good idea. How often depends on how many partners you have and the type of sex you have.

* Most gay men choose to go to a GUM clinic for a health check. It is easy to find out where they are in your area from the Internet (see Further Information, Resources, Website and Organisations, page 263).

* During a visit you will be offered screening for all STIs, usually including HIV.

* If you receive treatment, always complete the course. Never share tablets and don't have sex until you are clear of infection.

* If you do have an infection, partners will need to be told. The clinic will help you with this.

* NSU, followed by gonorrhoea, are the most common STIs in gay men.

* Outbreaks of syphilis have been reported among the gay communities in London, Brighton and Manchester – most often picked up and passed on through oral sex.

* STIs are not necessarily a sign that a sexual partner has been playing around. Herpes and warts can appear many months after first catching the infection.

* At GUM clinics you can be vaccinated against hepatitis A and B.

* You can prevent the spread of HIV by using condoms for anal sex.

* It is possible to pick up HIV by performing oral sex on an infected man, especially if he ejaculates in your mouth – but the risk is lower than from unprotected anal sex.

* A treatment called post-exposure prophylaxis (PEP) may protect you if you have been exposed to HIV through receptive unprotected anal sex. This is usually available from GUM clinics or hospital accident and emergency departments, but treatment must start within 72 hours of exposure.

* There are now good treatments for HIV that can slow the virus down.

SYMPTOM CHECKER

If you think you have contracted an STI you should get a health check-up. The following checklist will help you identify a possible cause of your symptoms but is no substitute for professional medical advice.

		Gon	Chlam	NSU	Herpes	Hepatitis	Syphilis	HIV
Penis	Discharge	+	+	+				
	Lumps/bumps							
	Blisters/sores				+		+	
	Pain when urinating	+	+	+	+			
	Itch				+			
Testicles	Painful	+	+	+				
	Lumps/bumps							
	Itch							
Anorectum	Discharge	+	+		+			
	Lumps/bumps							
	Blisters/sores				+		+	
	Pain when defecating	+	+		+			
Throat	Discomfort when swallowing	+	+					
	Swollen lymph nodes ('glands')				+		+	
Faeces	Pale					+		
	Diarrhoea							+
Body	Rash				+/-	+	+	+
	Feeling weak					+	+	+
	Fever				+	+	+	+
	Itch					+		
	Lumps/bumps							
Eyes & skin	Yellowish					+		

183

		Crabs	Scabies	Gut infections	Warts	Molluscum
Penis	Discharge					
	Lumps/bumps	+	+		+	+
	Blisters/sores					
	Pain when urinating					
	Itch	+	+			
Testicles	Painful					
	Lumps/bumps	+	+		+	+
	Itch	+	+			
Anorectum	Discharge					
	Lumps/bumps				+	+
	Blisters/sores					
	Pain when defecating					
Throat	Discomfort when swallowing					
	Swollen lymph nodes ('glands')					
Faeces	Pale					
	Diarrhoea			+		
Body	Feeling weak			+		
	Fever			+		
	Itch		+			
	Lumps/bumps				+	+
Eyes & skin	Yellowish					

FOURTEEN

PENIS PROBLEMS

Sexually transmitted infections (STIs) are the most common cause of problems affecting the penis but there are others, ranging from bending and breaks, to problems with the foreskin. Gay guys can have high expectations of themselves and put a lot of emphasis on their sexual ability. But being able to perform at the 'flip of a switch' is something that only occurs in porn films – not in real life. Yet many guys still judge themselves on the basis of their last erection and so if it doesn't work the way it should anxiety levels can rocket. In this chapter I'll work through some of the most common problems that guys have with their penis.

FORESKIN PROBLEMS

If your foreskin is red, swollen and itchy then you have what is medically known as balanitis. The foreskin can also be painful and difficult to pull back, or it may be cracked, making urinating painful. Balanitis is usually caused by fungal infection but can be due to infections such as herpes and syphilis or an allergy to soaps or shower gels. A fungal infection can also affect the head, or glans, of your penis, and can cause small red spots and/or a scaly rash.

Your doctor will probably be able to tell the cause of your balanitis just by looking but may take a swab specimen from the area just to make sure. Fungal balanitis is by far the most common cause and is easily treated with antifungal cream, which your doctor can prescribe. If your penis is painful, try bathing it twice a day in weak salt water. If your doctor thinks that the problem is caused by an allergy or sensitivity to soap then just use water to clean the area and the inflammation should settle.

Once the infection has cleared up, keep your penis clean by regularly washing under the foreskin with clean water, as this can prevent it happening again (see page 53). Frequent attacks of balanitis can cause scarring and tightening of the foreskin (phimosis, see below), and may require removal of the foreskin (circumcision).

Other skin problems such as eczema and psoriasis can affect the foreskin and head of the penis. Your doctor can prescribe creams and ointments that can help.

PHIMOSIS AND PARAPHIMOSIS

Phimosis, the condition in which the foreskin is too tight to pull back, can reduce your enjoyment of sex because you can't expose the sensitive head of your penis for stimulation. It can also be painful when you become erect, as the head of your penis can get trapped inside your foreskin. Some men find that they can make the foreskin more flexible by lubricating it thoroughly and then slowly stretching it. But usually the only solution is circumcision (see page 52). Paraphimosis is where your foreskin gets trapped behind the head of the penis and you can't pull it forward again. Paraphimosis is very serious as it can cut off the blood supply to your foreskin. If this happens to you, get medical attention immediately.

'I'm really worried about my dick. I've got lots of white bumps at the bottom of it just above my balls. I can sometimes pop them. I've also got some strange-looking tiny finger-shaped things on the head of my dick.

I think they have been there forever and when I get hard they're more obvious. I just don't like the look of them.' Lucas, 24

There are times when there is nothing wrong with your penis at all but you may notice something that you hadn't noticed before. White bumps at the base of your penis are the hair follicles (cavities in the skin that house the hair roots). Sometimes they have hairs coming out of them and sometimes they don't. If you gently squeeze them – especially when they are soft, after a hot bath – they can pop and a small amount of white cheesy material will come out. Most guys have some at the base of their penis but they can also be found further up the shaft. Hair follicles can't be removed but knowing they're normal should make them easier to live with. Finger-shaped bumps around the edge of the head of the penis are called papules. They are entirely normal and typically stand out more when you get an erection.

BENDS IN THE PENIS

'I had a perfectly straight cock until about eight months ago. Then one day, without warning, it changed shape. It now bends forward about two inches from the top. It can be painful now and then but generally I can still have good sex with my boyfriend. I must admit, though, that it has affected my confidence.' Mario, 38

It is not unusual to have a penis that isn't completely straight when hard. Most times a curve causes no problems at all. But if your curve causes pain when you're having sex, or you find anal sex difficult, you could have a condition called Peyronie's disease. This is more common after the age of 40 and tends to come on slowly over a year or so.

The cause is not really understood but is thought to be the result of the penis being bent at an awkward angle, for example during penetration. This can cause scar tissue to build up on the lining of the penis. You can usually feel this as a thickening just below the skin. The penis then curves towards the direction of the scar when it becomes erect. The problem tends to run in families so there may also be a genetic cause.

In most cases, Peyronie's disease doesn't need treatment and does clear up naturally. But if the problem is interfering with your sex life you should see your doctor. Steroid injections, creams containing Vitamin E and surgery have all been tried but unfortunately there is no very effective treatment as yet.

PERMANENT ERECTION

The medical word for an erection that won't go down is priapism. It means that all the blood that has gone into making the penis hard has become trapped and can't escape again. This can not only be very painful but can also be dangerous because fresh blood can't get in and so your penis is starved of oxygen.

Priapism can happen at any age and to anyone. But it is more common in guys who have the blood disorder sickle cell disease and in men who inject their penis to treat erection problems. Antidepressant drugs and recreational drugs such as cocaine and ecstasy are known to cause priapism, especially when used in conjunction with Viagra or other 'anti-impotence' drugs that guys use to enhance erections. It can also be caused by cock rings that are left on too long or are too tight to remove.

Priapism is a medical emergency. Don't wait around! If it happens to you or to someone you're with then get help at once – especially if it lasts more than two hours. Without treatment there can be permanent damage to the tissues of your penis, causing impotence. Priapism is treated by draining the penis of blood and using drugs to shrink down the blood vessels.

ERECTION PROBLEMS

'Sometimes when I'm fucking a guy I find it difficult to stay hard once I'm in. It's been coming on over the last year and happens more when I'm with a guy for the first time. I want to try Viagra to see if that helps but I also like to take poppers and I've heard that the two together can be a problem.' Tom, 29

Having a problem with your erection is more common than you might think. Overall about 1 in 10 guys (10 per cent) will have a problem with his erections at some point in his life. The older you are the more likely it is to happen. Around 2 in 5 guys (40 per cent) who are in their forties can have erection problems. This rises to 7 in 10 men (70 per cent) who are in their seventies.[1]

The reality is that every man has times when he can't get an erection when he wants to or gets an erection but it just doesn't last the course. At times like that the problem is usually due to 'performance anxiety'. The fear that you won't perform actually inhibits your ability to have an erection.

If you start to have erection problems on a regular basis, or find that you get an erection but it's not hard enough or doesn't last long enough to have sex, then you may have what doctors call erectile dysfunction. The word 'impotence' is reserved for when you have the problem practically all the time.

For a long time, any problem a guy had getting an erection was regarded as psychological or accepted as a normal part of ageing, but this view has changed. Now we know there are both psychological causes and physical causes of *erectile* dysfunction. In 3 out of 4 cases overall (75 per cent), the cause is physical – especially in older men. In the case of young men, the cause is most likely to be psychological. Physical factors rarely operate alone because they will often affect your confidence, making the problem worse.

The following are the most common causes of erectile dysfunction:

Poor blood flow to your penis

The most common overall reason for erectile dysfunction is narrowing of the arteries that supply the penis. The penis can't then fill with enough blood to get erect.

The larger blood vessels to your lower stomach and pelvis can also be affected. If you smoke, have high blood pressure or diabetes this is more likely to happen to you.

Damage to the nerves that supply the penis

This can happen following spinal surgery or after an accident. Illnesses such as multiple sclerosis also affect the nerve supply to the penis.

Drugs

Recreational drugs such as cocaine, cannabis and alcohol can all inhibit your ability to get an erection. Prescription drugs to treat high blood pressure, indigestion or depression are also known to cause erectile dysfunction in some men.

Hormonal causes

The male hormone testosterone has a central role in sexual function. It gives you your sex drive – or libido – and is needed to get your penis hard. Low testosterone is a rare cause of erectile dysfunction in younger guys but is more common in older men because hormone levels naturally decrease as you get older. Men who use anabolic steroids also run the risk of having erection problems.

Psychological problems

Psychological or emotional problems can easily affect your ability and desire to have sex. They are thought to be the cause of erectile dysfunction in about 1 in 5 guys (20 per cent). Performance anxiety is often a factor – especially in young men. Worrying about whether you will be able to have an erection is a sure way of not getting one as the anxiety you feel inhibits your ability to get hard. And if it has happened once, then next time the worry that you won't be able to keep your penis erect and hard enough is so much on your mind that the problem is more likely to happen again. You're then caught in a vicious circle of worry and erection failure.

Underlying relationship problems are a common cause of erectile failure and so should be explored. Sex between guys can be full of potential psychological difficulties and many guys go through times when they feel guilt or shame for what they like and enjoy doing. This can affect their ability to get and maintain an erection.

Depression, stress and tiredness are all reasons why you might go off sex and for your erection to fail. It can be that your mind is more focused on work worries, or what needs doing round the house, than on sex.

Physical or psychological?

Finding the cause of your problem can sometimes be difficult. Your doctor will help you but you could also try answering the following questions to see what is the more likely cause. Often there is a mix of both physical and psychological factors.

How did it start? If your problem has come on gradually then a physical cause is more likely. Do you smoke, have high blood pressure or diabetes? Psychological causes usually come on suddenly, after some emotional upset or erection failure. This often leads to performance anxiety. Stress, depression, anxiety, and relationship, work or financial problems can all occupy the mind and have a knock-on effect, reducing your sex drive and inhibiting your ability to have sex.

Are you taking prescription or recreational drugs? Recreational drugs, and especially alcohol, are a common cause of erectile problems and so this is a good reason to give up or cut down. Tell your doctor if you suspect that the prescription drug you are taking is responsible, as you may be able to switch to one that does not have this side-effect. However, bear in mind that the underlying condition you are being treated for could also be to blame.

Do you get an erection at night or wake up with one in the morning? Erections usually happen about three to four times a night, usually during REM (rapid eye movement) sleep when you are most likely to be dreaming. Most men also wake up with an erection in the morning. If you have an erection when you wake up, this makes a physical cause less likely (but doesn't rule it out) and makes a psychological problem the more likely cause. If your morning erections are getting weaker over time this might point to a physical cause.

Can you get erect and ejaculate on your own - but not with a guy? If everything is working okay when you're alone but not when you're with someone it's more likely there is an emotional or psychological cause.

Do you cycle? Research shows that guys who spend hours in the saddle restrict the blood flow to the penis. They can also feel numbness because cycling compresses the nerves in the area too. If you're on your bike for less than three hours a week and you have a good-quality saddle this shouldn't be a problem.

What you can do

Gay men have a reputation for always being 'up for sex', so admitting you have a problem is difficult. The ability to have sex at any time and for as long as possible can be part of the 'perfect' gay image. So when you don't meet your own expectations, no matter how false they are, it can put a big dent in your self-confidence. Many men are too embarrassed to ask for help, yet the problem can have a big impact on their lives, often leading to anxiety and depression. Don't be embarrassed – you are not alone!

Perhaps even more important, the problem can be a warning sign of an underlying condition, such as diabetes or heart disease, so it's important to seek medical advice.

When you see your doctor, be honest about the problem. You'll be asked questions such as those listed above and you'll need to be examined. The doctor may arrange blood tests, to check for diabetes and possibly testosterone levels, if your sex drive has been affected. Because erection problems can be an early sign of heart disease, you may have your cholesterol checked as this can clog your blood vessels. Sometimes more specialist tests, for example, to check the blood supply to and from your penis, are carried out, if necessary.

The good news is that there are now good treatments for both physical and psychological causes of erection problems. Almost every man can be helped.

PHYSICAL TREATMENTS

There is a wide range of drugs and mechanical devices that can help you. The aim of treatment is to give you both a firmer erection and one that lasts long enough for you to enjoy sex. Everyone has heard of drugs such as Viagra (sildenafil), which has been around since 1998. But not everyone can take this type of drug. For example, men who take nitrate medications for heart problems may not be suitable. You and your doctor together must decide which is the best treatment for you.

Before discussing these medications it's worth remembering that even simple lifestyle changes, such as giving up smoking and taking regular exercise, can definitely help improve your erections.

Sildenafil (Viagra)

This is a drug you take in tablet form about an hour before sex. The usual dose is between 25 mg and 100 mg. At the moment it's only available on prescription for those with specific health problems such as diabetes, or disorders that affect the nerves. But a hospital specialist can prescribe it for you if your erection problems are affecting your day-to-day life.

How does it work? Viagra widens the blood vessels that feed your penis, allowing more blood in. But you still need to be turned on for it to work – it doesn't give you an erection by itself, as many guys still think. So it's not so useful if you've gone off sex. Most guys who take it get a firmer, longer-lasting erection and have a better chance of ejaculating. You take it about an hour before sex and the effect can last up to eight hours. If you eat a fatty meal it can delay the drug working.

Are there any problems? Like all prescriptions drugs there can be side-effects. Headache, skin flushing, heartburn or nasal congestion happens in up to 1 in 5 guys (20 per cent) who takes it. Some guys get altered vision and see shades of blue.

Tadalafil (Cialis) and vardenafil (Levitra)

Cialis and Levitra are newer tablets that work in the same way as Viagra. The usual dose is 5–20 mg of Cialis or 10–20 mg of Levitra, taken about an hour before sex. Like Viagra, these drugs are only available on prescription unless you have a medical condition, such as diabetes, or illnesses that affect your nerves, or you are seeing a hospital specialist.

How do they work? As with Viagra, these drugs widen the blood vessels that supply your penis, so when you are aroused more blood can enter, making your erection harder and longer lasting. They work for most guys. The effects of Levitra last for up to eight hours but Cialis sticks around in the body for longer and works for up to 36 hours in some guys.

Are there any problems? Similar to Viagra, these drugs can produce mild side-effects, such as headache, skin flushing, heartburn or nasal congestion. But this is rare.

WHEN SILDENAFIL, TADALAFIL AND VARDENAFIL CAN BE DANGEROUS

Many gay guys use Viagra in combination with other party drugs. Sales on the black market are huge.

Viagra and some other drugs, such as poppers (amyl nitrite), can make a deadly combination. So never take the two together. This is because both drugs dilate (widen) the blood vessels and so can lower your blood pressure to dangerously low levels. You should not use Viagra if you take nitrates, or other heart medications prescribed by your doctor. If you have heart problems, always check with your doctor before taking it.

Apomorphine hydrochloride (Uprima)

This is a tablet you put under your tongue 20 minutes or so before having sex. The usual dose is 2–3 mg.

How does it work? This treatment acts on the nerves in the brain that control your erection. It works for about 1 in 2 guys who uses it.

Are there any problems? The drug can cause mild side-effects, such as dizziness, headache and nausea. You shouldn't use it if you have heart problems.

Alprostadil (Muse)

This drug usually comes as a pellet that you place in the top of your urethra. It is simple to use. The packet includes a device that you slide into the top of your urethra that pushes out the pellet. You then massage your penis for a minute until the drug is absorbed into the tissues. Alprostadil is also available as a gel that you rub on your penis, or as an injection (Caverject and Viridal Duo). The injection, directly into the shaft of the penis, sounds pretty dramatic but it really does help – especially for those who can't take other treatments or who haven't responded to them. Some men find this difficult but you will be shown how to do it and it gets easier with practice. About 10 to 15 minutes later your penis will be hard and the erection lasts for about an hour. The injection works for 9 out of 10 men (90 per cent) who use it.

As with other drugs for erectile dysfunction, alprostadil is available on prescription for those with specific health problems, such as diabetes or illnesses that have affected the nerves. A hospital specialist may prescribe it for others whose erection problems are affecting day-to-day life.

How does it work? Alprostadil widens the blood vessels in the penis to increase the blood flow. This helps you to have a firmer and longer-lasting erection and so a better chance of orgasm. It works for most men who try it.

Are there any problems? A few men who use the pellet or gel get an aching pain in their penis when they use it, but there aren't any serious side-effects. Alprostadil *injections* can make the penis ache and there may be bruising at the site of the injection. For about 1 in 20 men the erection doesn't go down, a condition called priapism (see page 188). If this happens you need to see a doctor immediately.

Yohimbine

This is a chemical extracted from the bark of the yohimbe tree in Africa. It comes in liquid or tablet form but is not available on the NHS so you can't get it from your doctor. It is available on the open market, but speak to your doctor before trying it, in case there are any reasons why it may be unsuitable for you (see overleaf).

How does it work? Yohimbine is thought to work on the part of the brain that controls your sex drive and can be effective if there is a psychological cause for your erection problems. Research shows that it works for up to 1 in 2 men (50 per cent), making him more interested in sex and giving him firmer and longer-lasting erections.

Are there any problems? You shouldn't take this treatment if you are taking anti-depressants or have heart, liver or kidney problems. The most common side-effects of this drug are headaches, feelings of anxiety and more frequent urination than usual.

MECHANICAL TREATMENTS

Vacuum pumps and penile rings

These are used by men who have erectile dysfunction as well as those who want to enhance their erections. Your doctor may recommend that you use a vacuum pump before trying medication. You can buy both the pump and penile rings at a sex shop or on-line.

How does it work? Firstly the penile ring is pulled down the shaft of the penis to the base. The ring has side loops to stretch it open until you get an erection. The cylinder of the vacuum pump is then placed over the penis and a handle on the end is worked to pump air out and create a vacuum that draws blood into the penis. The ring is then closed around the penis to stop the blood leaving, so keeping the erection firmer for longer.

Are there any problems? Prolonged use of rings can damage the sensitive spongy tissue inside the penis. Rings can also squeeze the urethra and some men find that this stops them ejaculating, but they can still have an orgasm. Rings should never be left on for more than half an hour and you should make sure you choose one that is the right size. Pumps for medical use usually come with a choice of ring sizes (see also page 129).

Surgery

There are surgical operations that can help men with erectile dysfunction, such as inserting special bendable rods or inflatable tubes into your penis. Doctors call these treatments penile prostheses. But these operations are less common nowadays as medical treatments are now so effective.

PSYCHOLOGICAL TREATMENTS

The reason you are having problems with your erection may be more to do with how you feel about yourself, or because you're having difficulties in a relationship. If so, talking therapies, such as psychosexual therapy, or counselling, may help. As well as talking through your problem, you may be given exercises, such as 'sensate focus' (see below), that you can try with a partner. If the problem is due to performance anxiety or your problems started suddenly after a bad sexual experience, you may also be given medication such as sildenafil (Viagra) to help boost your confidence and get you back on track. Some men have found yohimbine useful in these situations as well.

Psychosexual therapy/counselling

This involves talking to a trained therapist/counsellor who can help you get to the source of your problem and then work through it with you. If you're having problems in your relationship then it can help if both you and your partner talk to the therapist or counsellor, both together and individually. Sensate focus is one of the most commonly used exercises and can help you to focus more on the emotional aspects of sex rather than concentrating solely on achieving an erection and orgasm. Sensate focus starts with a 'ban' on full sex and instead you both spend time touching and massaging each other – initially with no genital contact. It's about learning to enjoy these simpler sensations and becoming confident that your body can react to them.

These exercises also help remove the pressure of feeling you need to perform, and can strengthen the emotional bond between two people. Over several sessions, you'll be encouraged to begin to involve the genitals, but stopping short of orgasm at first, until the therapist/counsellor believes you are ready to go all the way. Exercises like these are easier if you are with an understanding partner. Remember, although only one of you may have an erection

I'M NOT UP FOR IT ANY MORE!

It's almost taboo in the gay world to admit that you are not 'up for sex'. But libido – or sex drive – varies from person to person. Some people just have a less powerful sexual urge than others. A mismatched libido can also cause problems in a relationship if one guy wants sex more often than the another. But just as couples disagree about other things in life, it's common to find couples disagreeing about how much sex there should be in their relationship.

You may find that you have less interest in sex now than you used to. Losing the desire to have sex is often a sign of being unhappy, stressed, tired or relationship problems. Stress can put a big damper on your drive – if you're more concerned with work issues then your mind is not going to be on sex. Low sex drive can also be a side-effect of illness, or prescription medication for heart problems or depression. Alcohol and recreational drugs also affect your drive. Rarely, a lower than normal level of the male hormone testosterone can also be a cause.

But there doesn't have to be a 'cause'. Sex drive reduces with age, in part because of lower levels of testosterone, but also because sex often becomes less of a priority and focus of attention. If you have been in a relationship for a while then it is common for your sex drive to decline unless you try to keep it fresh, for example through 'sex exploration' (see page 123).

Finding the cause of low sex drive is very similar to that of erection problems. Possible physical causes need to be looked at, along with any emotional problems or issues.

problem, the root cause may be the relationship itself and so both of you need to be willing to find a solution.

If you're single, you can feel even more anxious because of the pressure to perform the first time with a new partner. Simple honesty can often help. Saying that you're enjoying the sex you are having but that you are nervous and so finding it difficult to get hard or cum can diffuse the situation. Even better, try to have a conversation before you start! If a guy rejects you, remember that's his problem – not yours. Sexual confidence comes from having a positive self-image, and so someone who is not prepared to put you at your ease and who undermines your confidence by rejecting you, just because you can't always perform on demand, is not worth knowing.

Psychosexual therapy can be difficult to get on the NHS but there are voluntary agencies that can help. For more information see Further Information, Resources, Websites and Organisations (page 263).

Erection problems can also sometimes be a symptom of depression. It's important to see your GP if you're feeling down. Treatments such as counselling can help and antidepressant drugs may be given as well. Unfortunately these medications also can affect your sex drive and ability to have an erection, and so are not always an ideal solution.

EJACULATION PROBLEMS

Sex can be full of anxiety. If the quality of the erection is the first concern for a gay man, then the second is with ejaculation, either 'cuming too soon' (premature ejaculation), 'finding it hard to cum' (delayed ejaculation), or 'not cuming at all' (anejaculation).

Premature ejaculation

Most guys have known a time when they've ejaculated too soon – usually just because they were too worked up. It's the most common of the ejaculation problems and affects about 1 guy in 5 (20 per cent) at some time. Like all sexual problems, it can affect how you feel about your life and relationships. Like other sexual worries, gay guys can have unrealistic expectations of themselves and think that they have a 'problem' when in fact everything is normal.

When having anal sex a man will usually ejaculate after three to five minutes of continuous thrusting. It's not the hours that porn films suggest or that your friends may brag about. So what exactly is 'too soon' or premature? There is no absolute definition but ideally you should be able to delay ejaculation long enough for your partner to enjoy sex as well.

What is the cause? Premature ejaculation is more common in younger guys, especially guys who haven't had much sexual experience. Sex is then very new and fresh so it's not surprising that control levels are not high.

There's usually no physical reason for premature ejaculation and a psychological cause is more likely. Some people think it is tied up with early sexual experiences. For example, it might be because you are used to having hurried quick sex (including masturbation), perhaps because you are frightened of being discovered, or you feel bad about the sex you have, and so subconsciously want to get it over and done with as quickly as possible. This can programme you to orgasm quickly even when you are in a different environment and at ease with yourself. Premature ejaculation can also be a sign that you're feeling stressed or unhappy in yourself or with your relationship – either sexually or emotionally.

What is the treatment? There is a special 'pause-and-squeeze technique' you can try and drug treatments that may help, but unfortunately there is often no quick fix.

✱ Pause and squeeze technique: This is an exercise to train your body to delay the desire to ejaculate and to 'step back' from an impending orgasm. You can practise this either when you masturbate or when you have sex with someone else. It does help some men but needs a little effort – as well as an understanding partner, if you're with someone.

　Once you get an erection, start masturbating or having sex up to the point when you think you might ejaculate, then stop! And don't give yourself any more stimulation for about thirty seconds. You or your partner can also squeeze the head of your penis where it joins the shaft. The sense that you are going to ejaculate should subside. Then, after the pause, start stimulation again, and again pause before you are about to cum. Do the whole cycle about four or five times. With time you'll be able to pace yourself and no longer need to stop or squeeze. If this is not working for you then psychosexual therapy could help. Your GP can refer you to a therapist.

* Topical treatments – local anaesthetics: There are sprays and gels that contain local anaesthetics. These work simply by reducing the sensation in the head of your penis.

* Tablets: Some antidepressants have the side-effect of delaying ejaculation. These tablets have not been licensed for use for premature ejaculation but many doctors are now prescribing them for the problem. So far research shows that taking a tablet on a daily basis or just three to four hours before having sex can increase the time before guys ejaculate from under one minute to more than three minutes.

BLOOD IN SEMEN

Although scary, blood in semen is usually nothing to worry about. During sex tiny blood vessels can easily get broken and cause a dramatic-looking streak of blood in your cum. It's more likely to happen after a session that was more vigorous than usual. But it can sometimes be a sign of an infection, or a problem with your prostate, or possibly high blood pressure, so it's worth seeking your doctor's advice.

Delayed ejaculation

'I have been with my boyfriend for about eight months and although we still have sex it take me ages to ejaculate, or sometimes I just can't. I do get an erection and get very excited, but that is how it ends. It's very frustrating!' Stefano, 24

Most men find that, occasionally, they find it difficult to ejaculate – often because they're just not in the mood, or have been having a lot of sex. Where there has been a change in your sexual performance, or where you have always found it hard to ejaculate when having sex, the underlying cause is most likely to be an emotional problem. Usually men with this problem find that they only have difficulties when they have sex with a partner, and when masturbating alone they are okay.

What is the cause? Sex between men can be full of emotional difficulties. If delayed ejaculation has always been a problem, it could be that on some level you find intimacy difficult or that deep down you're not completely comfortable with your sexuality and the fact you're having sex with men. If it is a recent change, it might be because you are tired, stressed, unhappy or unsure about who you are with. All these factors can affect how relaxed you are during sex and stop you really 'letting go' – something that is essential for you to orgasm. Unfortunately, once you start to worry about your difficulty in ejaculating it is likely to make the problem worse next time. Of course, it can be that you're not being turned on enough, or not getting what you want from sex or from your partner.

There are some physical causes that need to be born in mind. Prescription medications, such as antidepressants, heart medications, or recreational drugs can also impede the ability to orgasm.

What is the treatment? Physical causes need to be ruled out first, so chat to your doctor about the problem. He or she may need to carry out a physical examination and may run some tests. If the cause of the problem is emotional, then talking about it with a partner can often help. It can also be useful to go back to basics. A first step is to be able to masturbate until you ejaculate with a partner just near you – but not touching you, as this may put you off. Next, allow some intimacy such as kissing while you masturbate. As your confidence builds, you'll be able to let him finish you off with his hand or mouth. You'll need your partner to give you his full support but with time most men with this problem are able to enjoy a full sex life.

Psychosexual therapists or counsellors can help you through these difficulties, too. You can be referred to one by your GP or you can visit a sexual health clinic.

However, the availability of these counsellors varies around the country. If you have a partner it is often better if you both go together.

The type of sex act that really brings men to a climax varies from one guy to the next. Some men respond and can ejaculate through oral sex, while others can only do so through anal sex. If you think it's simply a problem of becoming aroused then only you can know what gets you going. It may be time to start asking for it. Have the confidence to live out your fantasies – and if your partner doesn't know how to do it the way you want, then show him. Remember that everyone is different and so has different preferences over the types of sex they enjoy. What turns you on will also change with time – so what worked in the past may not work today.

KEY POINTS

* Fungal infections can make the foreskin red, swollen and itchy. It is easily treated with an antifungal cream, available from your GP.
* One in 10 men has a problem getting an erection at some point in his life.
* There are good medications for erection problems that help most men.
* Don't self-treat if you have a problem – see your doctor for a check-up.
* Talking therapies (psychosexual therapy/counselling) are useful when there are emotional or psychological reasons for erection problems.
* Premature ejaculation can be treated with medication or sex techniques.
* Delayed ejaculation usually has an emotional or psychological cause and is best treated through psychosexual therapy/counselling and/or sexual exercises.

FIFTEEN

TESTICULAR PROBLEMS

Sexually transmitted infections (STIs) can affect the testicles, as well as the penis, because the infection spreads up from the urethra. But there are some specific disorders that only affect the testicles and these will be dealt with in this chapter along with problems and solutions relating to semen (or 'cum').

PAINFUL TESTICLES

'I've got really big balls and sometimes they ache. I had them checked out and there is nothing wrong with them but still every now and then they can be painful. So I'm kind of living with it. It was a relief to know that it wasn't something nasty like cancer.' Adam, 31

Epididymo-orchitis

This condition is an inflammation of the epididymis (the tangle of tubes that sits above and behind each testicle) and one or sometimes both testicles. In younger gay men, it is usually caused by an STI, such as chlamydia or gonorrhoea. In men over 35 it tends to be due to a bladder infection. However, it can also be caused by minor injury – say by not wearing underwear or through cycling or gym training.

The main symptoms are pain and swelling of the testicles. If the infection is in the epididymis alone then only this part will be tender. The skin of your scrotum, or testicular sac, can look red and feel warm. You may also feel unwell and have a high temperature.

If it is due to an STI, you may have other symptoms, such as discharge from the penis and a stinging pain when you urinate.

What should I do? This condition needs urgent medical attention. Visit your GP or a GUM clinic. You will need to have swab specimens taken from your penis to identify any infection. If one is found, antibiotic tablets can cure it provided they are taken as soon as possible after you develop symptoms. Some guys leave it far too long and end up in hospital needing antibiotics given straight into a vein through a drip or may even need surgery to remove the infected testicle. Epididymo-orchitis can be very painful, so wearing supportive underwear can also help and you'll need to take pain killers.

When mild inflammation of the epididymis (epididymitis) is from a minor injury, taking anti-inflammatory painkillers such as ibuprofen should help and you could also try wearing something a little more supportive for a while.

BLUE BALLS

The dull pain or mild ache that some guys get when they've spent too long getting aroused and have not had an orgasm is called 'blue balls'. This is because the scrotum can look a little blue because it is starved of fresh blood. The ache will die down naturally after a few hours without any treatment, but if you have an orgasm the relief will be immediate!

SUDDEN PAIN IN THE TESTICLES

'About three weeks ago my left ball became very painful – I mean serious pain! I've never felt anything like it! I was at home, so thought it would just get better by itself but by the afternoon I couldn't bear it any more. I finally got seen at A&E and I was rushed to theatre. They said my ball had twisted and they had to take it out. If I'd gone earlier then they might have been able to save it.' Zac, 19

Sudden pain and swelling in the testicles can be due to a testicle becoming twisted, a problem called torsion. This twisting cuts off the blood supply and starves the testicle of oxygen. It is more common in guys under 25. Torsion is very painful and can also make you feel nauseous or even vomit. Your testicle is so sore that you can't bear it being touched!

If this happens to you, don't wait around. You'll need to have a small operation to untwist the ball. If the testicle stays twisted for more than four hours then permanent damage is likely and you'll have to have the whole testicle removed.

LUMPS AND BUMPS

It's a good idea to examine your testicles from time to time (see page 63) to check for problems. The most serious potential problem is cancer of the testicle, called testicular cancer, but there are lots of other less serious problems too.

Testicular cancer
This is the most common cancer in guys aged between 15 and 35. Each year there are about 1,400 cases in the UK, so it's really important to make sure you know about this.[1] Thankfully, it's a cancer that can be cured in most men. But it must be diagnosed and treated as early as possible.

It is not known why some men get testicular cancer and others don't. But it is more common in men who had an undescended testicle when they were young. This is a problem found in babies in which a testicle, which is inside the abdomen in the foetus, fails to descend into the scrotum before birth. If it doesn't descend normally after birth then surgery is usually necessary.

What are the symptoms? The main symptom of cancer of the testicle is that one testicle feels bigger than the other. You may also feel a lump in your ball. There is not usually any pain but some men say the testicle felt heavier or ached. Rarely, the cancer can spread to other parts of the body and cause symptoms including backache, cough or breathing difficulty.

What should I do? If you feel that a testicle has changed in size or shape or you feel a lump in your testicles that you're unsure about, it's always best to see your doctor for an examination. You may find this embarrassing but that won't compare to the way you'll feel if you leave it till it's too late. Your doctor will probably send you to have an ultrasound scan of your testicles to check for any lumps. The ultrasound scan uses sound waves to produce an image of the testicle.

What is the treatment? If tests show that you have cancer there is a very good chance that you will be completely cured. You will need to have the affected testicle removed through surgery – but this is not a major operation. Sometimes chemotherapy or radiotherapy are needed if the cancer has spread to other parts of your body.

Having one testicle will still allow you to enjoy a full and active sex life. One testicle can supply all the testosterone you need – and sperm, if being fertile is important to you. After treatment you can have a fake testicle put in, for cosmetic reasons.

Varicoceles, cysts, hydroceles and hernias

'I checked out my balls with my boyfriend and my sac just feels different to his. My testicles feel okay but in the stuff beside them I can feel a couple of hard lumps the size of peas.' Richard, 20

There are many other types of lumps and bumps that men can have in the scrotum. One of the most common findings when guys examine themselves is a varicocele. This is a swelling of the veins that runs from the top of your testicles into your body. These blood vessels can stretch and dilate (widen), causing what are basically varicose veins. Doctors often describe them as feeling like worms. You can sometimes see the swelling of a varicocele just under the surface of the skin of the scrotum, more often on the left side than the right. Varicoceles can cause fertility problems because they make the testicles warmer than they should be, which isn't good for sperm production. Usually varicoceles don't cause any symptoms but some men feel an ache on the affected side. If fertility is important to you or your varicocele aches then a small operation can fix this. However, as with all operations, there is a slight risk of infection and, for unknown reasons, it doesn't always get rid of the ache.

Another lump you may feel is an epididymal cyst. These are usually small pain-less firm lumps that you feel in your epididymis – the coils of tubes behind each testicle. No treatment is needed for these. They are just harmless bumps and cause no symptoms so they can be left alone. But remember, always get your doctor to check any lump you find.

A hydrocele is another kind of lump on the testicles. It is a collection of fluid that can form around one testicle and is completely harmless. Doctors can usually tell the difference between a hydrocele and a tumour by shining a light against the lump. The fluid in a hydrocele reflects a reddish colour, whereas a solid tumour does not reflect light at all. Unless it is very large, a hydrocele does not cause any problems and so does not need any treatment. If it is large, it can be drained of fluid.

A final lump that you can feel in your scrotum is a hernia. It is more common in older guys. A hernia occurs when part of the bowel pushes through a hole in the abdominal muscles. In younger guys it can happen from lifting heavy weights, which can strain the abdominal muscles and cause them to weaken. The small loop of bowel squeezes through the hole, and is felt as a swelling in the groin. Sometimes the loop of bowel can get pushed all the way down into the scrotum and cause a swelling there. A hernia should never be ignored. The intestine can get twisted or trapped, which may block the blood supply, a condition called strangulated hernia, which needs emergency treatment. A small operation may be needed to push the hernia back inside the abdomen and then the hole in the abdominal muscles is closed.

KEY POINTS

* If your testicles are painful see your doctor. You may have an infection, which needs medical treatment.

* In young men, such infections are usually caused by sexually transmitted diseases that have spread to the testicles from the penis.

* Get into the habit of checking your testicles regularly for lumps and bumps.

* Testicular cancer is the most common cancer in guys aged between 15 and 35 and can be cured if found early.

* Most other lumps and bumps in the testicles are harmless and need no treatment but should still be checked out by your doctor.

SIXTEEN

ANORECTAL PROBLEMS

'I love getting fucked but my current boyfriend is a big lad. We've tried to go slow but the day after we did it last week it was really painful to have a shit. I didn't notice anything at the time – but I suppose I was quite worked up! Things seem to be settling now, but I wonder what damage I – or he – did!' Brian, 30

Your bottom is one of those areas where you can't easily see what's going on. This often adds to the sense of panic you feel when something isn't right. Thankfully, most problems here are not serious and are easily sorted out.

Many guys think that if they see their doctor about any problem to do with their arse they are going to have to 'out' themselves because they think it must be due to anal sex. Even if they don't have anal sex, they worry the doctor will think they have! Most problems relating to the anus can and do happen to any guy – gay or straight – and aren't always connected to anal sex.

PILES (HAEMORRHOIDS)

If you notice bleeding after you've opened your bowels, you most likely have piles, or haemorrhoids. Piles are swellings of the delicate veins of your anus and rectum. These can be 'internal', in which case they are inside your anus so you can't see or feel them, or 'external', in which case you can feel them as soft lumps around the rim of your anus.

Piles are very common – about half the UK population has had them at some time, so you are most definitely not alone. Anal sex doesn't cause them! The most common cause is constipation and having to strain to push the faeces out. They are also linked to being overweight and lifting heavy weights. All these put pressure on the delicate veins in the anal canal, causing them to stretch and swell. Piles are basically varicose veins of the anus. They bleed when craggy, hard lumps of faeces scrape past when you open your bowels or from being bashed during anal sex.

What are the symptoms? Piles may cause discomfort but are usually painless, and so you'll only know you have them when you notice some bleeding after you've been to the toilet. They can sometimes be itchy or cause a discharge of mucus. You'll see fresh blood on the toilet paper or in the bowl. If your piles are large and close to the anal opening you can feel them outside your anus. If you have piles you may get some bleeding after having anal sex.

Rarely, a blood clot (thrombosis) can form in a pile. You'll feel this as a firm lump on the edge of, or just inside, your anus. If you take a look at it (using a hand mirror) it will look like a bluish grape. This type won't usually bleed but is usually, although not always, extremely painful. It usually takes about ten days for the blood clot to be reabsorbed into the body. After that you'll be left with a small skin tag on the edge of your anus.

What is the treatment? If you do notice some bleeding from your anus there are treatments that can help. Many of these you can get over the counter from the chemist, but some are only available on prescription from your GP. It can be best to see your doctor so you can be checked for rarer causes of bleeding too. It's best to avoid anal sex while your piles are still bleeding to give them time to heal.

Treatment is with creams, ointments, or suppositories – large tablets you put inside your rectum. A widely used brand is Anusol. Most contain a local anaesthetic that will ease the pain. Some contain a corticosteroid (hydrocortisone) that can reduce inflammation, but you'll need to see your GP to get these because they are only available on prescription. You'll usually need to use these treatments for up to a week before the inflammation settles completely.

For an external pile that has developed a blood clot (thrombosed), you can reduce the swelling by placing ice packs wrapped in a kitchen towel against your anus, and painkillers can help ease the pain. But check the packet ingredients and avoid any painkillers containing codeine, as these can make you constipated, which will only worsen the situation. Painkillers that contain paracetamol or ibuprofen only are best.

Sometimes the anal sphincters can go into spasm, which is very painful. Sitting in a warm bath can relax the anal sphincters and ease the pain. If it's a big thrombosed pile, a small operation is usually needed to remove the blood clot. The pain relief from this small procedure is immense. Removal of the whole pile is sometimes recommended, too, so that you don't run the risk of it happening again.

The most important treatment for your piles is to keep your stools soft, by eating lots of fibre and drinking plenty of fluids, and avoid straining on the loo. This will help the bleeding and discomfort settle and, hopefully, the problem will not happen again. If you don't do this then going to the toilet will be very painful.

Prevention: Protein can make up a large part of a gay man's diet, but it can also make you constipated. To avoid this, your diet needs to be high in fibre – fruit, vegetables and wholemeal bread are all good sources – and make sure you drink extra water. For example, you could have an apple or banana with that post-workout protein milk shake. Fibre supplement drinks, which you can get from any pharmacy or from your GP, can help, but it's better to try to get all the fibre you need from your diet. Regular aerobic exercise, such as walking, jogging, and cycling, also helps prevent constipation.

When it comes to opening your bowels, make sure you pay attention to your body. Go to the toilet when you feel the urge, and don't hold it back, because this will lead to the build-up of larger and harder stools that are more likely to cause problems. When you do go to the toilet, don't strain and don't just sit there for ages reading your latest copy of *Boyz*, as this makes it more likely that you will strain.

Recurrent piles: If you're having a lot of problems with your piles, there are other treatments that can help. For these your GP will need to refer you to a hospital specialist. Banding (tiny elastic bands that are placed around the piles to make them shrivel and drop off) or injections into the piles are the most common treatments. Both are painless and don't need general anaesthetic. If the problem is more serious, you may need an operation under general anaesthetic to remove all the piles.

INCONTINENCE

'I worry that if I get fucked a lot I'll not be able to shit properly. I'm a bottom but worry that I'm doing permanent damage to myself.'
Antonio, 22

Some guys worry that if they have lots of anal sex they'll end up being anally incontinent (not being able to control their bowels). Anal sex does stretch the anal sphincter muscles, so it's common to have an occasional accident, especially the few hours after sex. But the anal sphincter muscles soon return to their normal size.

If you are into large sex toys or fisting, it is possible, but very rare, for the internal sphincter muscle to become permanently lax. This could then cause problems with bowel control later on. To reduce the risk of damaging your sphincter muscles, always allow time for them to relax completely before anal sex, using toys or being fisted. Toning your anal sphincter muscle through Kegel, or pelvic floor, exercises can also help (see page 65).

ANAL FISSURE

An anal fissure, a tear in the lining of your anus, is usually caused by passing large hard stools, but may also be caused by anal sex, fisting or using sex toys. These activities can also make a tear worse.

What are the symptoms? An anal fissure causes a severe, sharp pain when you go to the toilet. The pain can even last for an hour or more after you have been to the toilet. Tears don't need to be very big to be painful. The area is supplied by thousands of nerve fibres so even a small tear can cause a lot of pain. The fissure may also bleed when you pass stools, but usually only a small amount.

What is the treatment? Most fissures will heal by themselves over a week or two. To ease the pain, creams or ointments containing a local anaesthetic that are used to treat piles can be used. Creams containing hydrocortisone can ease inflammation and are available through your GP.

As with piles, keeping your stools soft is really important or going to the toilet will be extremely painful. Eat plenty of fibre and drink plenty of water. Your GP can also give you medication to soften the faeces. It is a good idea to see your doctor if you think you have an anal fissure as the symptoms can be similar to anal herpes infection. Anal sex will be painful at this time so it's best to avoid it until the tear has healed. To help ease the pain caused when the sphincter muscles go into spasm, you could try sitting in a shallow warm bath.

If an anal fissure was caused by sex, then try to work out why it happened so it doesn't happen again. If you've had one fissure you have a greater chance of having another because the wall of the anus is weaker at the point where you had the tear. The most common reasons for damage during sex are using too little lube, not giving your anal sphincters time to relax or using dildos or being fisted. If you have a lot of pain then it's a good idea to get a medical check-up because a bad tear may even need surgery.

When a fissure does not heal: For a few unfortunate men, anal fissures either fail to heal completely or do heal but then easily tear again. Sometimes an ointment containing glyceryl trinitrate (GTN) helps to aid healing. This relaxes the anal muscles and dilates the blood vessels in the area, bringing more blood, nutrients and oxygen to speed tissue repair. Botox injections can stop the muscles contracting and so give the fissure time to heal. Rarely, a small operation is required to reopen the fissure and allow it to heal again.

PERFORATION

A potentially fatal, but thankfully very rare problem that is more likely to happen during fisting or when using sex toys is a perforation, or puncture, of the lining of the rectum. It is less likely with anal sex because, unlike a dildo, the penis is softer and less likely to break through the delicate mucous lining. If this happens you may feel pain immediately. But if the tear is small or you are high on recreational drugs, you may not feel any pain initially. However, the pain will get worse, especially if any faeces escape through the tear, causing an infection inside the abdomen. Along with the pain, you'll then feel feverish and very unwell. A perforation is a medical emergency requiring a stay in hospital and a course of antibiotics given directly into a vein. Very rarely, surgery may be needed to remove part of your bowel. For more advice on how to fist and use sex toys safely, see pages 118 and 126.

PROSTATITIS

'I think that I'm not ejaculating with the same force that I used to. It used to be a very strong spurt, but it's weaker now. I've also got some discomfort between my balls and anus when I cum.' Felix, 28

Prostatitis is inflammation and swelling of the prostate gland. It can be caused by an infection but often a bug is never actually found. Prostatitis is a common problem and affects about 1 in 2 men (50 per cent) at some point in his life. It's not linked with being gay. The condition can cause a wide range of symptoms, which can sometimes make it hard to diagnose.

Prostatitis is split into two types, depending on how long your problems have lasted.

Acute prostatitis

When the condition comes on suddenly and makes you feel very unwell it is called acute prostatitis. This is usually due to an infection. In younger men it's most likely to be caused by a sexually transmitted infection (STI), such as chlamydia, that has spread to the prostate from your urethra. Sometimes putting objects down your urethra can introduce other types of bacteria that can infect the urethra and spread to your prostate. In older men acute prostatitis is usually a result of a bladder infection, and could be a sign of an enlarged prostate. This can constrict the urethra, preventing the bladder emptying properly, causing an infection that spreads to the prostate.

What are the symptoms? Common symptoms are:

* Pain or aching in your testicles, perineum (the area between your testicles and your anus), rectum, lower abdomen or lower back.
* Blood in your semen and/or urine.
* Urinating more frequently.
* Discomfort when you urinate.
* Difficulty urinating.
* Discharge from the penis.
* Fever and general aching – this may be a sign that the infection has spread through your body.

What is the treatment? If you have these symptoms, get medical help straight away. Prostatitis can be a very serious illness if the infection spreads into your bloodstream. The doctor will examine you by inserting a gloved finger into the anus to feel for the prostate. A urine sample will be checked to identify the bacterium responsible. Usually a course of antibiotic tablets taken for a couple of weeks will clear the infection but serious cases may mean admission to hospital for a few days to receive antibiotics through a drip straight into a vein.

Chronic prostatitis

If you have recurring problems with your prostate, or your acute prostatitis lasts for a number of months, it is called chronic prostatitis. Unfortunately this is often a difficult problem to treat.

The most common cause of chronic prostatitis is a condition called chronic pelvic pain syndrome. Doctors aren't sure what causes this but it's not thought to be due to an STI. It is thought that it may be due to a problem with the muscles that surround the prostate gland or with the structure of the prostate gland itself causing recurrent infections.

What are the symptoms? Usually, men with this problem have had symptoms for a number of months. The most common ones are:

* Pain behind the testicles, or at the end of your penis, when you urinate or ejaculate.
* Urinating more frequently, or an urgent need to urinate.
* Blood in the semen.
* Erection problems and lack of sex drive.

How is it diagnosed? Chronic prostatitis can be difficult to diagnose and you'll probably need to see a specialist for tests. These can include tests on your urine and blood, and swab specimens taken from the end of your penis.

What is the treatment? If an infection is found to be the cause of your chronic prostatitis, antibiotics can help. You usually have to take these for a number of weeks. Masturbation is recommended on alternate days to stop the prostate getting congested with a build-up of fluid.

If your problem is thought to be due to chronic pelvic pain syndrome, treatment can be more difficult. There is currently no single treatment that can cure this problem. Drinking plenty of fluids to stay fully hydrated can help. Doctors usually recommend that you ejaculate a few times a week to clear your prostate.

Antibiotics may be used and painkillers can be taken to ease any pain. New and more specialised treatments are being developed all the time and your specialist will be able to discuss these with you. In future there may well be a better outlook for guys with this problem.

Chronic pelvic pain syndrome can have a dramatic effect on your life. It is linked to feelings of depression and other psychological problems, which may also need treatment. You may be reassured to know that this syndrome is not life-threatening and you can't pass it on to someone else through sex. In about 1 in 3 men, the problem clears after about a year but for many the problem lasts much longer.

ITCHY ANUS

Having an itchy anus is a surprisingly common problem. And one that can be embarrassing to see a doctor about.

Most commonly it is due to an allergy or sensitivity to soap or shower gel, or irritation from substances in the faeces, such as spices, coffee, alcohol, milk products, fruit acids or even vitamin supplements. All these can make the skin around your anus red and cracked and very itchy – especially at night. You can react to these substances at any time, even if they have not caused a problem before. Common skin conditions such as eczema and psoriasis can also affect this area and an itchy anus can also be a symptom of syphilis, gonorrhoea, scabies, and threadworms (see Chapter 13). Piles are, however, rarely the cause of an itchy anus.

The treatment will depend on the cause. An STI or threadworms will require specific treatment. If these are ruled out by your doctor then an allergy or sensitivity is the most likely cause. Avoid highly scented soaps, bath oils or creams around your anus and try cutting out likely foods and drinks. A weak steroid cream from your GP or pile cream will also soothe the area and dampen down inflammation.

RASHES AROUND THE ANUS AND GROIN

The anus and groin area is naturally quite airless and sweaty. This makes it a breeding ground for fungal infections and so can cause a red itchy rash around your anus, or around your testicles and inner thighs, called Tinea cruris. It can be treated with an antifungal cream available over the counter from the chemist or from your GP. Always follow the packet instructions, but in general you should apply the cream to the rash and a few centimetres beyond it twice a day. Carry on using the cream for a few days after the rash has gone, to ensure that the fungus has been completely cleared. If a cream does not work then an antifungal tablet may be needed. You would need to see your GP for this as you cannot buy it over the counter.

Keeping your groin and the area around your anus clean and, importantly, dry can prevent fungal infections. Change your underwear daily and especially after playing sports or gym training. Using talc can also help and don't share towels as you could pass on the infection to someone else.

KEY POINTS

* Most problems related to your anus can affect any man – gay or straight – and so won't 'out' you to your doctor.
* The most common complication following anal sex is bleeding. The most likely underlying cause is piles.
* A cream or suppositories are usually all you need to treat piles. You can get these from your GP or from any chemist.
* The best way to prevent piles is to have a diet high in fibre and avoid straining when you open your bowels.
* A painful and bleeding anus is likely to be caused by a tear in the lining, called an anal fissure.
* An anal fissure can heal naturally but as that part of the anal wall has been weakened it is more likely to tear again.
* Prostatitis causes a dull ache behind your testicles.

* Prostatitis is usually caused by an STI and so needs prompt treatment to prevent the infection spreading to your bloodstream.
* An itchy anus can be due to infection or a skin problem such as eczema or psoriasis, but often it is caused by sensitivity to soaps, or bath oils, or to certain foods.

SEVENTEEN

SEX ADDICTION

Sex addiction or sexual compulsion is defined as having constant thoughts of sex and not being able to control the impulse to have sex.

It's true that gay men can have and enjoy lots of sex. Surveys of guys on the scene show that just over 1 in 10 men (10 per cent) has more than 30 partners a year.[1] Being addicted to sex isn't about having a lot of sex with lots of different people. It is a sign that you have lost control over your sexual urges and can't stop having sex no matter how hard you try.

The signs of sexual addiction are:

* Being unable to stop having sex, no matter what the consequences.
* Needing more and more sex to be satisfied.
* Craving high-risk sex and so putting your health in danger.
* Using sex and fantasy as a way to cope with stress or problems.
* Spending long periods of time looking for, having, or recovering from sex.

You don't become a sex addict over night. Often men go from one type of addiction to another, perhaps starting with compulsive masturbation when young to an obsession with magazine or Internet pornography. The Internet is fast becoming a source of addiction. Many men easily spend hours on-line every day and one study of gay men shows that up to 3 per cent of respondents using gay Internet sites said they were addicted to them.[2] It could be that the growth of the Internet and access to such a wide range of pornography is actually increasing the number of men getting hooked on sex in general.

Men who are addicted to sex often tell of losing touch with friends, and spending much more than they can afford on sex chat lines, pornography or escorts. They may have been arrested or cautioned for having sex in a public place, and are more likely to go to risky places for sex such as saunas or cottages. Addiction to sex often goes hand in hand with alcohol abuse and taking other recreational drugs.

What effect does sex addiction have?

The addiction can be so strong that all your energy is taken up in the pursuit of sex. As a consequence, sex addiction often has disastrous effects on relationships – being unable to commit to, or stay with, one person – as well as on finances, and home and work life. The sex addict's lack of control puts his health at increased risk from sexually transmitted infections (STIs) because his desire for sex is so strong.

Why am I addicted?

There are many reasons why someone develops an addiction to sex. For some it's related to low self-esteem and so it becomes a way of feeling wanted or needed. Others use sex as a way to escape from dealing with emotional problems. Research also suggests that men who are addicted to sex are more likely to have been sexually abused or emotionally abandoned in the past.

What is the treatment?

Just like other addictions, if you think that you might have a problem there is help available. The best treatment is talking therapy. This is available through your GP who will refer you to a psychosexual counsellor. Working through your problems and discussing how you feel about sex with a trained therapist will help. You'll also learn ways to change your behaviour and build your confidence.

Many men feel anxious about seeing their GP. Thankfully, there are excellent voluntary organisations that can also help you. They often use similar techniques used to help with addictions to alcohol or other drugs (see page 263 for further information).

At times depression can go hand in hand with sex addiction. Again, talking therapies help as can anti-depressant medications.

KEY POINTS

* Sex addiction is defined as having constant thoughts about sex and being unable to control the impulse to have sex.
* It can go hand in hand with other addictions.
* Sex can be used as a way to deal with or avoid emotional problems.
* Being addicted to sex usually leads to risky sexual behaviour and a greater chance of picking up and passing on STIs, including HIV.
* The good news is that there are talking therapies available that can help people who are addicted to sex.
* The hardest step is admitting you have a problem and seeking help.

PART V
DRUGS

EIGHTEEN

DRUGS: SAFER USE AND ADDICTION

'Most of the guys I know do drugs. I never used to but since I started going out clubbing you just kinda get involved and feel that as everyone else is using them it's the thing to do. I love the buzz, but I hate the come-down. The week after, we all say never again! But, of course, a couple of weeks later we do it all again.' James, 24

Whatever you feel about drug taking, drug use is widespread in the gay community. One recent study of almost 15,000 gay men across England showed that 1 in 4 had taken class A drugs in the last year.[1] But it's not just about illegal drugs. Alcohol, smoking and anabolic steroids are just as popular, if not more so.

Recreational drugs damage your health. In the short-term, many speed up your pulse, putting excessive stress on your heart, and raising your blood pressure – often to dangerous and possibly lethal levels. Drugs in your system are broken down by your liver, which has a vital role in keeping your blood clean. Too much drug use, too often, and you risk seriously damaging your liver, possibly leading to long-term problems. The breakdown products from the liver are filtered out by your kidneys, which can also be put under strain as well. Taking drugs also weakens your immune system, and this, combined with not eating properly and not getting enough sleep, can leave you wide open to colds and viral infections.

> *'I've never done drugs and I don't want to start. All those guys – if only they could see themselves when they're high – their eyes popping out of their heads, sweating and grinding their teeth. Not pretty! They give gay clubs and gay guys a bad name – that we all take drugs and can't have a good time without them.' Gordon, 29*

Recreational drugs can make you feel good, boost your confidence and help you lose your inhibitions. This makes it easier to meet and chat with other guys. They also make you feel sexy, and horny, and can enhance sexual pleasure. But their effects are short lived – unless you take more and more. When they do finally wear off, your brain is left short of essential chemicals. The after-effects, or 'come-down', can leave you feeling anxious, paranoid and depressed for a lot longer than the high you felt while you were on them. Your sleep pattern and appetite are often affected, too, so this can add to your overall feeling of ill health. If you suffer from depression or anxiety then they are likely to make you feel even worse in the long run.

SAFER RECREATIONAL DRUG USE

There is no completely safe way to take recreational drugs. Not only is there a danger to your health but most are illegal so you run the risk of arrest, fines and/or imprisonment with all the potential negative consequences that can have on your family, friends and career. If you are going to take drugs then there are measures you can take to reduce the risk to your health. That includes knowing the potential problems if you go overboard.

* Some gay men use drugs for sex because it gives them the confidence to explore their sexuality when otherwise they might have feelings of guilt over what they like to do. But it can get to the stage where they can't have sex without drugs. Plus, there is plenty of research to show that guys on drugs are more likely to have risky, unprotected sex, which puts them at greater risk of contracting a sexually transmitted infection and HIV. The sex that guys have when taking drugs also tends to be more aggressive or more adventurous. Drugs deaden pain sensations so what can seem like a pleasurable pounding will leave you bleeding and in pain the next day. In addition, drugs can have the opposite effect, making it impossible to have an erection or simply putting you to sleep!

* Many gay men don't take just one drug but often two or three together to make a cocktail of drugs. It should be obvious that the more drugs you take, the more often you take them, and the more you mix them, the greater your chances of serious problems. Some drugs taken together, for example GHB and alcohol, can be lethal. Again, if you feel you *must* use drugs, try to take them only occasionally, by themselves, and in moderation.

* There can be a lot of peer pressure on the scene and it's natural to want to fit in, so those who say they will never try drugs often end up changing their minds – or having them changed. If it is not your thing then have confidence in your decision. Remember that you are an individual – you don't have to run with the herd.

* Drugs not only change your mood to a great extent but usually also exaggerate the way you are feeling. So if you are already feeling anxious or depressed, avoid them – they will only make you feel worse, if not while you are on them then definitely afterwards, when you come down.

* If you have an ongoing condition such as epilepsy or a heart disorder it is best to avoid taking drugs as they could interact with the medication you are taking and make your health problems worse.

* When you are high with your friends make sure you all stick together – don't let anyone just wander off. It goes without saying that taking drugs alone is more risky. You know that your behaviour will change on drugs so try to set some limits on what you do – and respect yourself.

* Drugs often raise your temperature and, together with dancing in a hot atmosphere, can make you sweat more and so lose fluid. Remember to take regular drinks to keep yourself topped up. But avoid alcohol as this will dehydrate you more, so choose sugary, non-alcoholic drinks. Don't take drugs and drive or accept lifts from guys who are on drugs.

* You should expect to feel depressed after a weekend on drugs. It is not you. It is the drugs that are making you feel this way, so be kind to yourself. Don't make any life-changing decisions, no matter how much you may feel tempted!

* Respect your body and give it time to recover after a night out. Eat well and drink plenty of fluids, avoiding coffee and tea, which will only dehydrate you more, and get enough rest to recharge your batteries.

DRUGS AND HIV

If you are HIV positive, taking drugs can be especially risky. The biggest one is that while you are high you are likely to forget or be unable to take your medications – often missing doses altogether. This poor adherence to your drug programme can let the virus become resistant to your medication. In addition, dancing through the night, and so not sleeping or eating properly, will do nothing but weaken your immune system.

There is also the effect of the drugs themselves. Most recreational drugs are broken down by the liver and some HIV medications, especially protease inhibitors (PIs), inhibit the liver enzymes that break down these drugs. This means that the drugs you take may attain much higher concentrations in your body than you might have expected, leading to more severe and potentially fatal side-effects. This doesn't happen with all drugs but is a particular problem with ecstasy and possibly GHB and crystal meth (see pages 252, 254 and 250). If you have HIV, don't use party drugs. If you decide you want to use them, speak to your HIV specialist first.

WHEN THINGS GO WRONG

Side-effects from drugs are common. If you start to feel unwell whilst on drugs, tell your friends and find somewhere quiet to go that is away from crowds. Different drugs have different side-effects. Keeping calm and being patient usually pays off, but if you feel very unwell get help. Don't self-treat and take other drugs to counter what you think you may have taken.

GETTING HOOKED – ABUSE AND ADDICTION

Despite horror stories, most guys take drugs without developing a serious problem. For many it is just a phase they go through or they reserve their drug-taking for odd occasions. While using drugs can seem fun and exciting at first, for most guys the excitement and pleasure they get out of it fades with time. It's common to get tired of that scene and move on. Partying becomes less of a priority or you start to feel more independent and confident in who you are and no longer feel the need to fit in.

However, about 1 in 4 gay men (25 per cent) says he worries about how much he drinks – and just over 1 in 5 (around 20 per cent) says he worries about his drug taking.[2] It is not always that easy to tell when you might be starting to develop a problem with drugs or alcohol. But there are warning signs to look out for that suggest it is time to stop and think about how much or how often you're taking them. These include the growing feeling that you're consuming too much drink/drugs, feeling guilty about how much you're drinking/taking, problems at home or at work, friends noticing a change in your personality, and getting into trouble with the police.

All recreational drugs are addictive up to a point. Some highly so, such as nicotine, alcohol, heroin and cocaine; some less so, such as ecstasy. Physical dependence is when you need more and more of a drug to get the same high, and get withdrawal symptoms when coming off the drug, and so feel compelled

233

to keeping on taking it. Psychological dependence is when you are unable to go out and have a good time without taking the drug. Addiction can affect anyone but is more likely if you have a relative who also has or had problems with addiction to drink and/or drugs.

Here is the crunch. It is when you realise that you have a problem that you have the best chance of changing your behaviour. Once you have accepted that you are not happy with what you're doing and that you have a problem and *want to* change, then change *can happen*.

If you think that you're taking more than you should, the first step is to try to cut down. It can help to avoid the places where you know you'll be tempted, and change your circle of friends. Don't try to change your whole life in one go as you're more likely to fail. Just try working on the drugs issue to start with. Once you've done that you can start looking at other areas of your life. Also look at the triggers that make you want to take drugs, drink or smoke. If stress is a cause, or you can only feel confident and relaxed when high, think of new ways to handle it or why you lack confidence.

No one will say that changing your behaviour is easy. You may miss the highs of the drugs you used to take and the social life that goes along with it. There is pressure in the gay world to stay where the action is, and keeping away from places and friends could make you feel isolated. Once you start to make changes you'll be surprised how good you feel. With time, your new habits will feel more natural than your old ones.

There is a lot of specialist help out there that can support you along the way. Getting support will make it much more likely that you will be able to change and maintain your behaviour. There are many groups and organisations that offer different types of help depending on your problem – some specially for gay men. You can have individual or group therapy and if you do get hooked on drugs then there are medications that can replace the drug and, with help, you can slowly work your way off them completely. See Further Information, Resources, Websites and Organisations, on page 263.

KEY POINTS

* Drug and alcohol use have always been widespread in the gay community.
* They alter the way you feel and think and make it more likely you'll have unsafe sex.
* What goes up always comes down – so after a drug 'high' you have a drug 'low' that often lasts longer.
* All drugs can harm your physical health.
* Being HIV positive makes drug taking even riskier. If you are on medication you may forget to take it, and some HIV medications boost recreational drugs to dangerously high levels in your body.
* If you are going to take recreational drugs, try to make taking them as safe as possible.
* Most men take a long time to realise and admit they have a problem with drugs. Once they do there is help available to kick the habit.

NINETEEN

DRUGS, HEALTH AND SEX

In this section I discuss the use of alcohol, anabolic steroids, tobacco and recreational drugs. These are the drugs that are most commonly used by gay men. As a doctor I don't condone drug use. But I know that some guys will want to take them, if only to discover 'what they're really like'. I therefore believe it is my job to give you the plain, unvarnished facts about drugs so you can decide for yourself. By knowing their effects, the risks they pose to your health, and how they can affect your sexual life, you are better able to make an informed decision about whether to use them or not.

ALCOHOL

The most popular drug by far. Because it is socially acceptable and readily available, alcohol is used on just about any occasion. It comes in a wide variety of forms – including beer, wine and spirits. After you drink alcohol, it is absorbed by your stomach and intestines into your bloodstream and then works its way to your brain. It takes about an hour for the liver to break down one unit of alcohol (that's half a pint of moderate-strength beer, one unit of spirits, or a small glass of wine). So the more alcohol you drink, the longer it stays in your system.

The ups

Alcohol dampens down those parts of the brain that keep a check on your behaviour, so you become less inhibited. Small amounts can make you feel relaxed, happy and more confident. It increases blood flow to the skin, so you feel warmer. And alcohol also enhances the mood you were in when you first started drinking, so if you were feeling upbeat before you had a couple of drinks you are likely to feel even more so afterwards. Of course, the opposite also applies, so if you were feeling down, alcohol can make you even more depressed.

The downs

Alcohol affects the motor centres in the brain that control speech and coordination. As you drink more your speech starts to slur, you become unsteady on your feet and feel dizzy. Carry on drinking and you can fall asleep – or unconscious – and because your breathing is slowed you may even fall into a coma. Vomiting when drinking too much is common. If this happens when you're asleep then it can go into your windpipe and have fatal consequences. Because alcohol slows nerve impulse you become less coordinated.

Alcohol needs water to be broken down and removed from the body. It also suppresses a chemical that controls fluid levels and so you pee more. This results in dehydration, and together with any toxins in the drink, is the main cause of your headache and hangover the next day. Because alcohol is a depressant drug it's usual to feel tired and even a bit depressed or flat after a night out.

Alcohol: sex and health

*   Alcohol is an anaesthetic so it is easy to injure yourself when drunk and not notice. If you're having sex you are also less likely to feel any pain.
*   Drink too much and you are more likely to have unsafe sex or sex that you'll regret. How many times has alcohol been the reason why you wake up in the morning thinking 'What have I done?'
*   And while alcohol can loosen you up – too much and you'll not be able to get it up.
*   Most people enjoy alcohol without any problems but it is potentially addictive. Regular heavy drinking can soon lead to the need to keep drinking.

★ Small, regular amounts of alcohol are good for your health. But if you drink more you are less likely to eat well, sleep well or exercise, and you can also put on weight. If you regularly go over the recommended limit – for guys, that's three to four units a day with two or three alcohol-free days – or binge drink (consume a large amount in one session) you're putting your long-term health at risk. Alcohol can damage your liver, your nervous system, and cause depression and sexual problems, such as impotence.

ANABOLIC STEROIDS

'I've done steroids about seven times. I like the way I look and it gets me loads of attention! But I suppose I am worried that I may be damaging my body. I've never had any blood tests or anything. I didn't really know about that. I also got a breast lump after the last course – but I got some tablets from a friend that seem to be helping.' Marcelo, 25

Body culture and gay culture often go hand in hand. For some, the pursuit of the perfect physique leads them to taking steroids. Research in several London gyms popular with gay men, that was carried out back in 2000, showed that 1 in 7 gay men (about 13 per cent) admitted using anabolic steroids in the previous year.[1]

Anabolic steroids are synthetic versions of the male hormone testosterone. 'Anabolic' means 'protein building' and this type of steroid increases muscle bulk when used in conjunction with body building exercises. (Don't confuse it with another kind of steroid – corticosteroids – which are anti-inflammatory medicines.) The most commonly used anabolic steroids are Sustanon 250, Winstrol (stanozolol) and Deca-Durabolin (nandrolone). They can be taken as tablets, but most guys who use steroids prefer to inject the drug straight into their muscles.

It's important that body builders don't go overboard on protein intake: excess protein can be harmful as humans cannot process the nitrogen in protein efficiently. Intakes of protein above needs cannot be stored and can lead to bone demineralisation. There is also a link between high protein, especially processed forms, and bowel cancer.

239

Deaths from steroid use are very rare, but there are well-documented side-effects from using them. So if you take them, or are planning to, be aware of the following before you make your decision. Anabolic steroids can cause:

* Hair loss and premature baldness.
* Greasy skin causing acne, especially on the back.
* Raised blood pressure.
* Increasing levels of blood cholesterol. This can clog your arteries.
* Increase in size in your heart muscle. This can lead to heart disorders.
* Testicular shrinkage.
* Increased sex drive while you are taking steroids followed by rapid decline once you stop.
* Mood changes. Typically guys feel moody, irritable, aggressive ('roid rage'), depressed or even suicidal.
* Liver damage. Steroids are broken down in the liver and can poison it.
* 'Bitch tits'. This is excess breast tissue that can grow during, but more usually after, taking steroids – a condition called gynaecomastia. Usually this excess breast growth disappears once hormone levels return to normal. But if they persist, anti-oestrogen tablets or surgery may be needed.
* Prostate problems. Taking steroids may increase your chances of developing prostate cancer later in life.

The risk of developing these side-effects will depend on how much and how often you take steroids. From research involving London gay men, nearly all those who took steroids (96 per cent) said they experienced some side-effects:[2]

* 1 in 2 guys (50 per cent) said his testicles shrank in size.
* 1 in 2 guys (50 per cent) had problems sleeping.
* 1 in 4 guys (25 per cent) felt depressed between cycles of steroid use.
* 1 in 5 guys (20 per cent) had high blood pressure.
* Overall, guys who took steroids were more likely to have had suicidal thoughts in the preceding six months compared to guys who didn't take steroids.

Most, if not all, of these side-effects are reversible once you stop taking the steroids.

Thinking through the alternatives

Some guys rush to take steroids without covering the basics first. It takes time and effort to attain muscle bulk. So, before considering using steroids, look at your training programme – are you training hard enough? Try training with a buddy or personal trainer.

What you eat is really important when it comes to building up. So look at your diet to see that you're eating right. As well as eating protein to build your muscles you need carbohydrates for the energy to allow your body to grow. Most guys training hard use protein supplements.

You can check out most fitness stores and websites for other supplements, such as creatine, that can aid growth and recovery after training. Taken properly they are not likely to damage your health.

Most guys who use steroids feel happier when they are looking 'buff' and are not concerned with the possible health risks. But before you take that decision, ask yourself why you want to use them and what your expectations are. It can be linked to low self-esteem, so just make sure you've thought it out. How do you think your life would be improved if you were bigger?

Be aware, too, that although steroids can build you up there is no magic involved – you still need to train hard and eat well or you'll get all the health risks but no gains. The ultimate effect will depend on your original body shape. Be realistic in what you expect steroids to do for you.

Reducing your risk

There are voluntary groups that can give you advice on safer steroid use (see Further Information, Resources, Websites and Organisations, page 263). If you are going to take steroids, then the following are a few of the ways you can reduce the risk of harm:

* Know your source and what you are buying. Check the labels and make sure that what you are taking looks legit.
* Use the correct technique when injecting steroids and never share needles as this puts you at risk of blood-borne infections such as hepatitis and HIV.
* The more you take and the more often you take them, the greater the risk of problems. Start with low doses, and don't mix brands.

* Give your body a regular break from taking steroids. The usual advice is that if you take steroids for, say, six weeks, then take a break from them for the same length of time or – even better – double that time, to let your body recover.
* Protect your heart as much as possible. Don't smoke, have a low-fat diet and take regular aerobic exercise, at least 30 minutes doing some, for example, brisk walking, jogging or cycling, at least three times a week.
* Have regular blood tests to monitor the effects that steroids are having on your body. I'd strongly advise the following – before and after your course: liver function tests, kidney tests, blood glucose and lipid (blood fats and choles-terol) profile. Your GP may do these for you but you will need to disclose that you are taking steroids.
* Check your blood pressure before and during your course to make sure it isn't rising to harmful levels.

SMOKING

Studies show that up to 1 in 2 gay men (50 per cent) smokes – a much higher proportion than among straight men – and lung cancer is also more common in gay men than in straight men.[3]

The active ingredient in tobacco is nicotine, which can stimulate the release of a naturally occurring chemical in the body, called adrenaline, that is usually released in response to stress, fear or excitement. But tobacco also contains a mix of hundreds of different chemicals.

But smoking is not just about nicotine. Many men enjoy the whole ritual of smoking and the fact that it is a social drug that can be shared with others. It's also still linked in many minds to a sense of rebellion or glamour.

The ups

Every time a smoker has a cigarette the nicotine in it triggers the release of a burst of adrenaline in the body that causes a short-lasting buzz and a sense of relax-ation. Concentration and energy levels can also be heightened.

The downs

Smoking is one of the worst things you can do to damage your health, and 1 in 2 smokers (50 per cent) will die as a result of his smoking. It is known to cause lung disease, lung cancer and heart disease. It ages your skin, making it grey and dull looking, and in later life you have a greater chance of becoming blind (because smoking damages blood vessels in your retina) and impotent (because smoking damages the blood vessels in your penis). Smoking also reduces your sense of taste, stains your teeth and makes you smell unpleasant. Yet still gay men smoke.

Smoking: sex and health

* Tobacco is a very addictive drug. It is both physically addictive, so that when you are not smoking your body starts to crave nicotine, causing symptoms such as irritability and sweating, and psychologically addictive, so you always reach for a cigarette at times of stress. Therefore it is all too easy to get hooked.
* Quitting smoking is one of the best things you can do for your health. Even in the short-term your health will improve. Give up for ten years and your risk of lung cancer and heart disease will fall almost to that of a life-long non-smoker. Many worry about putting on weight but this risk can be reduced by eating a healthy, balanced diet and taking more aerobic exercise.

In the end, it comes down to really wanting to stop. Here are some tips that have worked for many people:

* Set a date and plan to stop completely. When you do, clear the house of anything related to smoking – lighters, ashtrays and, of course, cigarettes! Many guys feel irritable or get headaches – especially in the first few days – and, of course, you are going to crave a cigarette. But these symptoms do get better over a couple of weeks.
* Try nicotine replacement. Nicotine patches, gum or tablets can help ease the cravings. They are available on prescription from your GP.
* Use special medication. A drug called bupropion (Zyban) can help you quit by reducing the urge to smoke. This is available on prescription from your GP, too.
* Get support. Your GP's surgery may run a 'stop smoking' clinic that you can join. The support of others will improve your chances of stopping.

* Change your routine. Avoid places where others smoke or where your guard might be lowered after a drink or two. It is a good idea to keep clear of your usual haunts for a couple of weeks to avoid these tempting situations. You can't smoke in cinemas, theatres, museums, art galleries and libraries, so go there instead.
* Keep busy. Now is a good time to catch up on jobs, take up a hobby, visit non-smoking friends and relatives you haven't seen in a while, and it will stop you thinking about smoking.
* Save the money. The cost of smoking just 20 cigarettes a day adds up to hundreds of pounds a year and will set you back several thousand pounds over a ten-year period. Put that money aside and save it up so you can treat yourself to something you've always wanted.

AMYL NITRITE (POPPERS)

Amyl nitrite (poppers) has been used by gay guys for years. It is a clear yellowish liquid that comes in a small screw-top bottle. Guys who use it usually take a big sniff straight from the bottle. When fresh it usually has a sweet smell but when stale it can smell more like dirty socks. It is sold in sex shops, on-line and in some night-clubs.

The ups

Amyl nitrite is a vasodilator. This means that it widens (dilates) blood vessels. About fifteen seconds after taking a big sniff, you will get a rush and feel dizzy, warm, light-headed and relaxed. This all happens because your blood pressure drops. The effect doesn't last more than a minute because your heart speeds up to get your blood pressure back to normal. Many say this rush heightens sexual pleasure and makes an orgasm stronger.

The downs

Many guys say they get a throbbing headache after using amyl nitrite, especially after repeated sniffs. Others say they feel sick, dizzy or may even black out because their blood pressure drops too low.

Amyl nitrite can irritate the skin and so it is possible to get a rash around the nostrils. It is also flammable – so don't smoke when you use it!

Amyl nitrite: sex and health

* As with many other drugs, research shows that gay men who take drugs are more likely to have unsafe sex. This puts them at risk of contracting and transmitting HIV and other sexually transmitted infections (STIs).

* Amyl nitrite relaxes the smooth muscle of the anus and rectum and so lots of guys use it for sex. But there is a risk that you will be unaware of any soreness or pain during sex and this increases your risk of internal damage and getting an infection.

* You can become tolerant to amyl nitrite if you use it regularly – say for two to three weeks. Some men get psychologically hooked on it and end up not being able to have sex without it.

* Amyl nitrite can lower your blood pressure to dangerously low levels so you should never use it if you are taking medication for a heart condition or high blood pressure. Using amyl nitrite with drugs such as Viagra can be fatal because both dilate your blood vessels and cause your blood pressure to drop so low that your brain is starved of oxygen.

* Early on in AIDS history, some doctors thought that amyl nitrite actually caused AIDS, because so many gay guys used 'poppers'. There was even some research linking poppers to Karposi's sarcoma (KS). But, like AIDS, KS is now known to be caused by a sexually transmitted virus. There is, however, some research showing that frequent use of amyl nitrite – over a weekend, for example – may dampen down your immune system for the next few days and so increase your risk of picking up an STI.

AMPHETAMINES ('SPEED')

Amphetamines – commonly known as 'speed' – can be obtained as an off-white powder wrapped in paper, like cocaine, or as small white pills. They are stimulant drugs with a structure similar to the brain messenger chemical (neurotransmitter) noradrenaline.

As a powder, speed can be spread into lines and sniffed through a straw, or rubbed on the gums, or a small amount can be wrapped in cigarette paper and swallowed (called a 'speed bomb').

The ups

Half an hour or an hour after taking it guys say they feel awake, full of energy, talkative, confident and happy.

The downs

Speed makes some people feel panicky and nervous. Many get a tight jaw, dry mouth and dilated pupils, they sweat profusely and their breathing rate goes up. They may find it hard to sit still, let alone sleep, no matter how tired they feel.

After taking speed, the 'comedown' is proportional to how 'high' you were before. You often feel irritable, anxious and depressed – for up to a couple of days. Speed also dampens your appetite so at a time when you should eat well to replace lost energy stores you don't feel like it.

Speed: sex and health

* You are less likely to make reasoned decisions when taking speed. This can lead you to taking risks over with whom, where or how you have sex. For some guys, their sex drive increases, while for others it decreases.

* Speed can cause psychotic symptoms. You may have delusions and believe things to be true when they're not. Usually these symptoms wear off once you come down. But regular use can lead to depression or anxiety problems or longer-term problems such as actual psychotic-type illnesses.

* Speed both increases your heart rate and raises your blood pressure. This puts a strain on your heart and can cause dangerous palpitations. Your temperature can also rise dangerously. Some guys have died from a speed overdose and the risk is greater if you drink alcohol at the same time.

* Speed can be addictive – usually a psychological dependence. Without it you'll feel depressed, tired and hungry. The more you take and the more often you take it, the greater the risk of becoming addicted. You can also become tolerant to amphetamines so the more you use the more you will need to use the next time to get the same high.

* Often only about 10 per cent of the wrap you buy is pure speed. It may be mixed with other substances such as ground vitamin C tablets or caffeine.

BENZODIAZEPINES ('BENZOS')

Benzodiazepines are a large group of drugs, that include diazepam or temazepam. They are prescribed by doctors for sleep problems or anxiety.

The ups
Benzos make people feel calmer and more relaxed and can help them sleep.

The downs
Benzos make you drowsy, forgetful and uncoordinated. When taken with other drugs, including alcohol, there is a risk of accidental overdose. If you vomit while unconscious you may choke.

Benzos: sex and health
* Benzos can make you feel much less inhibited and less able to judge a situation correctly. This makes it more likely that you'll have sex when otherwise you might not, or have risky sex.
* Sex crimes have been committed through the use of a related drug, benzo rohypnol. If your drink is spiked you can go into a paralysed stupor, becoming unaware of where you are and therefore unable to prevent a sexual assault. Beware of accepting drinks from strangers unless you see them being served, and don't leave your drink unattended.
* Benzos are addictive if you use them regularly – both physically and psychologically. Your body can get used to them and you need higher and higher doses to get the same effect. If you do get hooked, the withdrawal symptoms can be very unpleasant, including heightened anxiety states and physical symptoms such as profuse sweating for a few weeks after stopping.

COCAINE ('COKE')

Cocaine (also known as 'coke' or 'Charlie') is a white powder that is extracted from the leaves of the South American coca tree. Lines of the powder are usually snorted through a straw or rolled-up banknote, or rubbed on to the gums. It can also be blown up the anus or mixed with water and injected.

The ups

Cocaine boosts levels of dopamine, the brain messenger chemical (neurotransmitter) responsible for some of the pleasurable feelings we experience. Cocaine makes you feel confident, sociable and full of energy. But the feeling can be so strong that it can verge on aggression and self-obsession.

The downs

What goes up must come down. Commonly, people who take coke say that, when they crash down from the drug, they feel irritable, anxious, sweaty, depressed or even paranoid, and don't sleep well. That's because the brain stops producing dopamine while you are high, leaving you running on empty until production starts up again.

The higher you were and the more you took, the worse you will feel when you come down. And the comedown will always last longer than your high – from a day to a week. Cocaine suppresses your appetite and so at a time when you need to eat to keep your system going you are not interested in meals.

The hit from cocaine lasts only about 30 minutes, so as the high wears off there is a strong urge to take more – coke is the number-one binge drug.

Cocaine: sex and health

* Cocaine is very addictive. The high is so intense it can be difficult to resist the urge to take it again. The main reason it is so addictive is that it prevents the re-uptake of dopamine in the synapses (gaps) where two nerve fibres meet. As a result, the dopamine receptors become exhausted and don't work at all. And tolerance happens fast – so the amount that got you high the first

few times is no longer enough, and you need to take more and more to achieve the same effect. If you become a regular user, you can soon find yourself seeking the drug just to prevent feeling low, anxious or irritable. What starts as a weekend treat can soon become a weekday compulsion – just to feel okay.

* Chest pains and even heart attacks are possible effects of regular cocaine use. The blood vessels of the heart become constricted, which reduces blood flow and forces your heart to beat faster and your blood pressure to rocket.

* Coke also causes irritation and bleeding of the mucous membranes of your nose. In frequent users it can even wear away the nasal septum, the wall of tissue that separates the nostrils. If you share banknotes or straws there is the possibility of contracting hepatitis B.

* Coke is an expensive party drug and regular use is likely to have a significant effect on your bank balance. Regular use can affect your ability to work or maintain relationships.

* Coke is often mixed with other drugs to pad it out – so you can never be sure what you are taking.

CRACK

Crack is the smokeable version of coke, made from cocaine, baking soda and water. It comes as small white lumps and is usually smoked in a small pipe. It can also be dissolved in liquid and injected. Its effects are similar to cocaine but stronger and shorter lasting. The cravings to carry on taking it are stronger, as is the comedown after using it. This all means that crack is far more addictive than cocaine. Take too much and it can be lethal, due to heart and breathing problems. Long-term use can lead to mental health problems such as anxiety and depression.

* While coke will often make you feel very horny and up for sex, your penis probably won't be. This is because the drug constricts the blood vessels supplying your penis and so reduces your ability to have an erection. Like most drugs, cocaine can affect your judgement and so there's a greater chance that you'll have unsafe sex and acquire – and pass on – STIs, including HIV.

CRYSTAL METH

Crystal meth (also known as 'Tina' or 'ice') has been around since the 1970s. It is a processed form of amphetamine (speed) and so is a stimulant drug. It comes as white rocks or crystals, hence the name, but is usually taken as powder and snorted like cocaine in small hits or bumps. Some guys rub it on their gums, swallow it in pill form, or inject it. Once it is in your system it causes the release of two types of brain messenger chemical, serotonin and dopamine.

The ups

Crystal meth is a powerful drug. Soon after taking a bump, guys say they feel high, clear headed and full of energy, and lose their inhibitions and become euphoric. The effect can last for hours. Users can stay awake for hours and often days.

A major effect of the drug is its impact on your sex drive – often turning the shyest man into a sex fiend. But, although the sex drive might be high, the drug often causes erection problems.

The downs

Users can become aggressive or even violent after taking crystal. And it is common to feel anxious or paranoid. The higher you go, the lower you will fall. What can be a high of your life can, a few days later, cause you to feel very depressed, aggressive, confused and even paranoid. Some guys get so low they feel suicidal.

Crystal: sex and health

* While on it, your blood pressure goes up, your body temperature can rise to dangerous levels, you can get irregular heartbeats and find it hard to breathe.

High blood pressure, which can cause bleeding inside the head, is the main risk and can result in strokes, paralysis and death.

★ Like cocaine, you can become addicted to crystal, with the added problem that you grow tolerant of its effects. So you need more and more to get the same high. Get hooked and it will have a major impact on your work and social life. The chances of you getting hooked are much greater if you smoke it in its purer form.

★ Compared to other drugs, crystal has the biggest impact on your chances of having unsafe sex. On crystal, your sex drive can rocket and the drug gets you so high you become unaware of pain and other warning signs. There are plenty of stories of men having rough sex where they are unaware of the damage they are causing themselves.

★ Long-term use of crystal can damage your brain cells. Regular use has also been show to cause permanent brain damage by killing the cells that make dopamine – similar to Parkinson's disease.

CANNABIS

Cannabis is probably the most widely used recreational drug, as shown by the number of names for it: 'spliff', 'weed', 'dope', 'hash', 'blow', 'draw', or it can be named after the place it comes from, such as 'Moroccan' or 'home-grown'.

It usually comes in resin form as a dark brown lump ('hash'), or as dried leaves ('weed'). Skunk is a purer and stronger form. Cannabis is usually mixed with tobacco and smoked in a joint or spliff. But it can be smoked alone in a pipe (or 'bong') or added to food or cakes ('space cake').

The ups

The effects come on quickly if you smoke it but may take up to an hour if you eat it. Most guys say they feel relaxed and happy. Some giggle for hours. It is a mild hallucinogen so it can enhance colours and the sound of music. Short-term memory loss is common and coordination is affected. The effects last for up to a few hours, depending on how much you take.

The downs

If you take cannabis when you're feeling down, anxious, or worrying about emotional problems, it's likely that you'll feel even worse. Some people can become agitated after smoking, or even paranoid, thinking that people are talking about them.

Other unpleasant effects are feeling sick or disorientated.

Cannabis: sex and health

* Cannabis raises your pulse rate, lowers your blood pressure, causes a dry mouth and stimulates your appetite (a symptom called 'the munchies').

* As far as the risks of lung and heart disease and cancer are concerned, smoking one joint is the equivalent of smoking about four cigarettes.

* It's not really possible to overdose on cannabis itself and it is not thought to be physically addictive. But the tobacco you use can be, and so some guys get into the habit of smoking it all the time and so become psychologically addicted. As a result they can't relax without a joint or can't sleep without having one. If you become a regular smoker you are likely to be less mentally alert than you would normally be.

* Cannabis has been linked to mental health problems, such as anxiety and depression, and more serious problems, such as psychosis, that may need hospital care. Usually, these symptoms improve if you stop taking it. But if you have mental health problems, such as schizophrenia or depression, then cannabis can make your condition worse.

ECSTASY ('E')

Ecstasy (or 'E') is one of the most popular club drugs. It became famous in the 1980s as the first 'rave' drug. Taken in tablet form, it is now often cheaper than alcohol. The active ingredient is MDMA, which stands for methylene-dioxy-meth-amphetamine. Like amphetamine, it mimics the action of the brain chemical dopamine. It can also come in powder form and is then taken by being rubbed onto the gums.

The ups

Men who take ecstasy say they feel a sense of warmth and euphoria. It's called a 'love drug' because it can make you more friendly and talkative and feel drawn to people. It also gives you the energy to stay dancing all night and makes you feel connected to the music. Some guys feel horny on the drug. The effects can take up to an hour to come on and can last up to eight hours.

Ecstasy can be a mild hallucinogen and you can experience distortion in sound and vision – especially if it has been mixed with other drugs such as LSD (lysergic acid diethylamide, or 'acid', see page 257) or ketamine (see page 256).

The downs

After taking it, the pupils of your eyes widen (dilate), your mouth becomes dry and you start grinding your teeth. Some say they feel anxious or confused while high. Many feel sick and may vomit.

Many guys experience a comedown in which they feel tired, irritable and depressed for a few days afterwards. They often find it hard to sleep for the next couple of days and night sweats are common. Appetite is also affected at this time.

Ecstasy: sex and health

* While taking the drug, your temperature rises dramatically, particularly when you are jumping around on the dance floor. You can easily become dehydrated because you are sweating so much and yet forget to drink or don't feel thirsty. Guys have died from taking ecstasy, either from overheating, irregular heartbeat, seizures (fits) or strokes.
* Taking ecstasy can also suppress your immune system, so in the days after a night or weekend taking the drug you are more likely to get colds or other infections or become generally unwell.
* As with many other drugs, while taking ecstasy you are more likely to have riskier sex. Yet for some men, although they want sex they can't get an erection.
* The long-term effects of ecstasy are not yet known. But there is some research that suggests long-term use may lead to mood and memory problems.

GHB ('G')

The full name of GHB is gamma hydroxybutyrate. The drug is also known as 'G' and there are several similar ones including GBL (gamma-butyrolactone) and butanediol. It is a powerful, quick-acting drug that usually comes as a colourless liquid with a slightly salty taste. It can also be in powder or capsule form. GHB is sometimes called 'liquid ecstasy', although it is in no way similar to ecstasy.

Although now illegal, the drug was first developed as a sleep aid. In the 1980s it was used by body builders because of a supposed ability to boost the release of hormones involved with muscle growth and fat reduction.

The ups

At lower doses, GHB acts as a stimulant. Within 15 minutes or so of taking a shot, the drug can make you feel happy and relaxed, as well as uninhibited and horny. The effects can last for up to a few hours.

The downs

At higher doses, GHB is a sedative and can make you feel dizzy and sick. Taking even more can lead to vomiting, sweating, muscle spasms and seizures (fits), and you may even pass out and can stop breathing.

It is very easy to overdose on this drug and it's very important to wait at least a couple of hours before repeating a dose because the drug builds up in the system. Just a tiny bit too much can push you over the edge into unconsciousness and needing emergency medical care. Most men who take the drug know someone who has been taken to hospital after taking too much. Many GHB *users* will suffer mild withdrawal symptoms, such as anxiety, insomnia and tremors, after a big weekend out.

GHB: sex and health

* As already mentioned, GHB makes you less inhibited and more horny – a dangerous combination. Guys on GHB are more likely to have unsafe sex,

254

putting you at risk of catching or passing on a sexually transmitted disease such as HIV.

* There are cases of guys being sexually assaulted after being given the drug unawares. Victims say they were aware of what was happening but were not able to resist.

* The big danger is that it is very easy to overdose on GHB. This can be life threatening and some have died. Most men who take it suffer some side-effects.

* Your body can develop a tolerance to it so that you need more and more to get the same effect. You can then become hooked or dependent on it. There are cases now of people who take it around the clock – when they stop they get withdrawal symptoms including anxiety, agitation, tremors and delirium – just as if they were coming off alcohol or benzodiazepine drugs ('benzos') such as valium. The long-term effects of taking GHB are not known.

HEROIN

Heroin is an opiate derived from morphine, itself derived from the opium poppy. Heroin has lots of names including 'gear', 'smack' or 'brown'.

In its purest form, it is a white powder but it is often mixed ('cut') with other substances and so can range in colour from white to brown. It can be smoked, snorted, or dissolved in water and injected straight into a vein. It is used by some guys as a 'chill out' drug, that they take to come down after an evening or weekend out on stimulant drugs.

The ups

Users of heroin say that just a few minutes after using it they feel a deep sense of calm and well-being and their life takes on a dream-like quality. Heroin is a very powerful painkiller, and can blank out both physical and emotional pain.

The downs

Heroin is highly addictive no matter how you take it. Soon users find their body needs the drug or they suffer severe withdrawal symptoms (called 'going cold turkey' or 'clucking') and feel sick, anxious, suffer muscle aches and have an intense craving to take the drug again. The body also becomes tolerant to the drug, so users need more and more to get the same effect. Once addicted, coming off the drug is very hard work.

Heroin: sex and health

* It is easy to overdose on heroin and deaths do happen, especially if it is mixed with other substances or used along with alcohol or benzodiazepines. Heroin can slow your breathing and heart rate until they stop altogether.
* Many people inject heroin into their veins, which then become swollen and inflamed and can get blocked, forcing users to find other veins around the body to inject into. Often users are forced to inject into their groin veins because the veins everywhere else have become so damaged. Injecting veins can cause severe infections.
* Sharing needles puts you at high risk of acquiring HIV and other blood-borne viruses such as hepatitis B and C.
* For many heroin addicts, their lives become completely dominated by finding and taking the drug. Their general health is neglected and the addiction can lead users into crime or prostitution in order to feed the habit.

KETAMINE

Ketamine, known as 'K' or 'special K', is a short-acting but powerful anaesthetic that is mainly used by vets when operating on animals but is sometimes used for humans as well.

It initially comes as a clear liquid but is usually baked to make a white powder that is taken in lumps ('bumps') like cocaine or crystal. It can also be injected – usually in the buttocks or other large muscle.

256

The ups

Guys say that at low doses ketamine makes them feel as if their mind and body have separated, as if they are floating above themselves – a sensation called disassociation. They move clumsily and have delayed sensations. This effect can last for an hour or two.

The downs

Some guys find the whole experience of ketamine very frightening. Too much and you will feel sick, vomit and go into what's called a 'K hole' where you can't work out what is going on, have great difficulty moving, develop symptoms of paranoia and feel completely separated from your surroundings.

Ketamine: sex and health

* Ketamine speeds up your heart rate and raises your blood pressure. Taken with other drugs that do the same thing, your blood pressure can rise to dangerous levels. In high doses, especially if you drink alcohol, your breathing may stop. Vomiting while unconscious on ketamine can lead to death by choking.

* As with most other drugs, you can become tolerant to it, so that you need to take steadily larger amounts to get the same effect.

* Some guys feel so turned on with low doses of K that they take more risks sexually than they would otherwise. The out-of-body feeling that some men describe can lead to a clouding of judgement when it comes to sex. Some men describe the sex they have as feeling as if it is not really happening to them. Again, this can lead you into doing things that you usually wouldn't that could put your health at risk.

LSD (ACID)

LSD stands for lysergic acid diethylamide, and is commonly known just as 'acid'. It usually comes as a tiny square of paper – often with pictures on it – but also comes in liquid or tablet form.

The ups

LSD is a hallucinogenic drug and so feeds off your imagination to give what's called a 'trip'. People who have had acid trips say that everything slows down and time is meaningless, their senses become heightened so that colours are more vivid and sounds are amplified. They experience hallucinations so that what they see and hear becomes distorted – and they become fascinated by mundane things such as the texture of paint. They may experience a distortion of senses so that they 'taste colours' or see their friends faces warp into someone or something else.

The downs

For some people, the experience of LSD can be very frightening – called a 'bad trip'. The paranoia, panic and confusion induced by the trip can be terrifying. The hallucinatory images that the mind generates can be nightmarish, for example, seeing the faces of people you know who are not really there, and it's possible to think negative thoughts about yourself or the world around you.

Trips usually last up to 12 hours and nothing can stop them – so, while they can be 12 hours of fun for some, they may be 12 hours of hell for others.

Acid: sex and health

* LSD doesn't heighten libido in most people – if anything it takes it away. It's not a drug that is linked with sex.
* The negative thoughts of bad trips have made some people attempt suicide. It is not possible to know in advance how LSD will affect you. But it is more likely that you'll have a bad trip if you are in a dark mood when you take it or are uncomfortable with the people you are with.
* Acid is not addictive but it can cause 'flashbacks' in which you relive part of the trip a few weeks, months or even years later.
* There are few reports of long-term health problems associated with taking acid, but if you suffer anxiety or depression it is more likely that you'll have bad experiences on the drug and that your anxiety and depression will get worse in the longer term.

MAGIC MUSHROOMS

These are naturally growing mushrooms containing hallucinogenic chemicals that have a similar effect to that of LSD. There are many different varieties that vary in their strength and the effect they have on the mind. People who take magic mushrooms either make a tea with them, or eat them raw, or add them to cooked food.

The ups

The effects of mushrooms are similar to LSD but usually milder. They usually come on about an hour after taking them and last for up to ten hours.

Milder varieties, or when taken at lower doses, can seem to slow the world down, heighten colours and make you feel relaxed and happy. Higher doses, or some stronger varieties, can have more powerful hallucinogenic effects and users have 'trips' similar to those on LSD.

The downs

Mushrooms can make you feel and be sick. What can seem like a lot of fun to one person can be a nightmare to another. Bad trips, just as on LSD, can be terrifying, with the user not knowing what is going on, feeling paranoid and being unable to prevent their imagination turning out strange images and distorted thoughts.

Magic mushrooms: sex and health

* Some magic mushroom varieties are poisonous so you have to be very careful that you make a correct identification before you eat any. Strength not only varies from one variety to another but may also vary in a single variety with the time of year, so it can be easy to take too much.
* Magic mushrooms are not addictive. But if you already suffer from anxiety or depression then magic mushrooms could make your symptoms worse.

KEY POINTS

* Possessing or supplying drugs is illegal and you risk a criminal conviction.
* Each drug has its potential ups – but, more importantly, its downs too.
* Before you consider using anabolic steroids to build muscles, look at alternative measures first, such as changes in your diet and training regime.
* If you do decide to take steroids, then have your blood and blood pressure checked regularly.
* Stopping smoking is the biggest favour you can do for your health.
* Amyl nitrite (poppers) can lower your blood pressure to dangerous levels if taken with Viagra or similar medications.
* It is possible to pick up and pass on hepatitis B through sharing banknotes when snorting cocaine.
* Overdosing on GHB is easy and can be fatal.

SUMMARY

You may have read this book from cover to cover or just dipped in and out for advice or ideas. However you have read it, I hope that you've found the answers you sought and picked up some new ideas about how to have better, more fulfilling sex while safeguarding your health. Everything we do in our lives carries a risk. So it is with our sexual and emotional lives. Not all risks and dangers can be avoided and sometimes it is necessary to take them – as in relationships – if we want to move on and develop. But we can also learn about how to avoid or reduce risks that may be harmful to our physical and psychological health.

I hope that through this book you can be more informed about how to balance those risks with your pursuit of a satisfying sexual and emotional life. If it has helped you at all then I'll consider my job in writing it worthwhile.

FURTHER INFORMATION, RESOURCES, WEBSITES AND ORGANISATIONS

Useful Organisations

Community HIV and AIDS Prevention Strategy (CHAPS)

www.chaps.org.uk

CHAPS is a partnership of community-based organisations, coordinated by the Terrence Higgins Trust, carrying out HIV health promotion with gay men in England and Wales. It offers advice, support and information on sex and sexual health, including counselling, outreach and workshops.

Families and Friends of Lesbians and Gays (FFLAG)

www.fflag.org.uk

FFLAG offers support and advice to lesbian, gay and bisexual people, and their friends and relatives.

Lesbian and Gay Switchboard

020 7837 7324

A confidential helpline helping with all lesbian, gay and bisexual issues, such as young people coming out, coming to terms with an HIV diagnosis or the loss of a partner. It aims to treat all callers with empathy, respect and compassion and acts as a source of information, support and referral for any issue relating to lesbian, gay or bisexual life.

National Aids Trust (NAT)

www.nat.org.uk

NAT is the UK's leading independent policy and campaigning voice on HIV and AIDS.

PACE

www.pacehealth.org.uk

PACE is an organisation that responds to the emotional, mental and physical health needs of lesbians and gay men in the greater London area, and offers counselling, groups and workshops on issues such as personal development, coming out, relationship skills, communication, sex and sexuality, HIV, mental health, eating disorders, spirituality, bereavement, assertiveness, alcohol and drugs issues, HIV prevention, employment, youth work and training.

Sigma Research

www.sigmaresearch.org.uk

Sigma Research is a social research group specialising in the behavioural and policy aspects of HIV and sexual health.

Terrence Higgins Trust (THT)

www.tht.org.uk

THT is the leading HIV and AIDS charity in the UK, and the largest in Europe. The website can help you to keep up to date with the law regarding the implications of passing on HIV to a sexual partner. It also has details of free, rapid HIV testing and of Terrence Higgins Trust publications.

Useful Websites

www.addictions.co.uk

A website set up to help deal with all types of addiction, including sex addiction.

www.aidsmap.com

This is a UK community-based charity organisation providing up to date information about HIV.

www.alcoholconcern.org.uk

Alcohol Concern is the national agency on alcohol misuse.

www.alcoholics-anonymous.org.uk
Alcoholics Anonymous.

www.bashh.org
For information on sexually transmitted infections (STIs) and HIV. Also use this website to help you find your nearest genito-urinary medicine (GUM) clinic for regular health check-ups, STI screening and other sexual health problems.

www.britishlivertrust.org.uk
The British Liver Trust for advice on Hepatitis.

www.cancerresearchuk.org
For information on testicular cancer.

www.drugscope.org.uk
Drugs information charity Drugscope: for information on the adverse effects and legal status of drugs.

www.freedoms-shop.com
This website is a good place to check out all the latest types and prices of condoms, even if you don't plan to buy on-line. Other websites for information on condoms include: www.bigboycondoms.co.uk *and* www.safex.co.uk

www.gaydar.com *and* www.gay.com
The two most popular gay dating sites. They enable you to view hundreds of profiles or search for your particular type in your city, county or across the world from the comfort of your own home.

www.gawhydontyou.com
This site features a massive directory of gay groups involved in sport, travel, cars – in fact loads that might interest you and help you meet other gay men with similar interests.

www.gayyouthuk.co.uk
This site features information and support for young gay people in the UK, including information and advice on coming out, including personal experiences.

www.gro.gov.uk
This government website gives information and advice on civil unions for same-sex couples, which give them the same rights as straight couples over issues such as inheritance, tax and visiting rights in hospital.

www.herpes.org.uk
Herpes Viruses Association: for advice, support and help about herpes infections.

www.metromate.org.uk
London based gay men's sexual health website offering information, courses and workshops, and links to other organisations.

www.norm.org
This website has information on the penis, including how to restore a foreskin after circumcision.

www.ocdaction.org.uk
For advice on body dysmorphic syndrome.

www.playingsafely.co.uk
An independent government-funded website which provides information on sexual health issues and sexually transmitted diseases.

www.queery.org.uk
This website provides listings for the lesbian, gay and bisexual communities in the UK and Ireland. The database covers the gay scene plus a wide range of non-profit services and non-scene community groups, as well as commercial business services.

www.sauk.org
Sexaholics Anonymous: a UK website helping with sex addiction.

www.ssha.info/public/index.asp
For information on STIs and related conditions.

www.sussedaboutdrugs.net *and* www.talktofrank.com
Two websites with advice and information on drugs and drug use.

Useful books

A number of authors, including Dr Stephen Goldstone, Daniel Wolfe and Terry Sanderson and Patrick Gayle have written excellent books on this subject that have provided me with inspiration.

The Gay Man's Kama Sutra, Kat Harding, Terry Sanderson (Thomas Dunne Books)

The Ins and Outs of Gay Sex, Stephen E. Goldstone (Bantam Doubleday Dell Publishing Group)

Men Like Us: The GMHC Complete Guide to Gay Men's Sexual, Physical, and Emotional Well-Being, Daniel Wolfe (Ballantine Books)

The New Males Sexuality – The Truth about Men, Sex and Pleasure, Bernie Zilbergeld PhD (Bantam Books)

The Ultimate Gay Sex, Michael Thomas Ford (DK Publishing)

REFERENCES

Part I: Gay Life

Chapter One: Being Gay

1) Troiden, R.R. *The formation of homosexual identities*. Journal of Homosexuality: 1989;17(1–2):43–73. Department of Sociology-Anthropology, Miami University, Oxford, OH 45056.

2) Sigma: *Time for more: findings from the National Gay Men's Sex Survey, 2000*. Sigma Research, 2001 (ISBN 1 872956 62 9). Ref 01C.

3) Johnson, A.M., Mercer, C.H. et al. *NATSAL: Sexual behaviour in Britain: partnerships, practices, and HIV risk behaviours*. The Lancet – Vol. 358, Issue 9296, 1 December 2001, 1835–1842.

Chapter Two: Coming Out and Finding Your Scene

1, 2) Sigma: *Out and about: findings from the United Kingdom Gay Men's Sex Survey, 2002*. Sigma Research, 2003 (ISBN 1 872956 71 8). Ref 03F.

3) Sigma: *'It makes me sick': heterosexism, homophobia and the health of Gay men and Bisexual men*. Sigma Research, 2005 (ISBN 1 872956 79 3). Ref 05A.

4) Sigma: *Out and about: findings from the United Kingdom Gay Men's Sex Survey, 2002*. Sigma Research, 2003 (ISBN 1 872956 71 8). Ref 03F.

5) Sigma: *Time for more: findings from the National Gay Men's Sex Survey, 2000*. Sigma Research, 2001 (ISBN 1 872956 62 9). Ref 01C.

Chapter Three: Cruising and Casual Sex

1) Sigma: *Risk and reflexion: findings from the United Kingdom Gay Men's Sex Survey, 2004*. Sigma Research, 2005 (ISBN 1 872956 81 5). Ref 05C.

2) Dodds, J., Mersey, D. *Sexual Health Survey of Gay Men, London 2004, Annual Summary Report*. Royal Free and University College Medical School, Department of Primary Care and Populations Sciences, Centre for Sexual Health and HIV Research.

3) Sigma: *Know the score: findings from the National Gay Men's Sex Survey, 2001*. Sigma Research, 2002 (ISBN 1 872956 64 5). Ref 02D.

4) Sigma: *Vital Statistics: Gay Men's Sex Survey, 2005*. Sigma Research, 2005 (www.sigmaresearch.org.uk/data05/All_England_2005.pdf).

5) Bolding, G., Davis, M. et al. *Use of gay Internet sites and views about on-line health promotion among men who have sex with men*. AIDS Care. 2004 Nov;16 (8):993–1001. City University London, Institute of Health Sciences, St Bartholomew School of Nursing and Midwifery, London.

6) Sigma: *Risk and reflexion: findings from the United Kingdom Gay Men's Sex Survey, 2004*. Sigma Research, 2005 (ISBN 1 872956 81 5). Ref 05C.

REFERENCES

Chapter Four: Relationships

1) Sigma: *Risk and reflexion: findings from the United Kingdom Gay Men's Sex Survey, 2004*. Sigma Research, 2005 (ISBN 1 872956 81 5). Ref 05C.

2) Sigma: *Time for more: findings from the National Gay Men's Sex Survey, 2000*. Sigma Research, 2001 (ISBN 1 872956 62 9). Ref 01C.

3) McWither, D. and Mathieson, A. (1996) 'Male couples'. In P. R. Cabaj and T. S. Stein (Eds) *Textbook of Homosexuality and Mental Health*. Washington, DC. American Psychiatric Press.

4) Sigma: *Out and about: findings from the United Kingdom Gay Men's Sex Survey, 2002*. Sigma Research, 2003 (ISBN 1 872956 71 8). Ref 03F.

Part II: Body Beautiful

Chapter Five: Skin, Nipples and Beyond

1) Sigma: *Out and about: findings from the United Kingdom Gay Men's Sex Survey, 2002*. Sigma Research, 2003 (ISBN 1 872956 71 8). Ref 03F.

Chapter Six: Cock

1) Sigma: *Know the score: findings from the National Gay Men's Sex Survey, 2001*. Sigma Research, 2002 (ISBN 1 872956 64 5). Ref 02D.

2) Wessells, H, Lue, T. F. and McAninch, J. W. *Penile length in the flaccid and erect states: guidelines for penile augmentation*. J Urol. 1996 Sep;156(3):995–7. Department of Urology, University of California School of Medicine, San Francisco, USA.

3) Mondaini, N., Ponchietti, R. et al. *Penile length is normal in most men seeking penile lengthening procedures*. Int J Impot Res. 2002 Aug;14(4):283–6. Department of Urology, University of Florence, Italy.

4) Wessells, H., Lue T. F and McAninch, J.W. *Penile length in the flaccid and erect states: guidelines for penile augmentation*. J Urol. 1996 Sep;156(3):995–7. Department of Urology, University of California School of Medicine, San Francisco, USA.

Part III: Sex

Information used in this section also from:

GMFA (Gay Men Fighting Aids) publications: *The Sex Course: What To Do with your Dick, Arse, Balls and Mouth. From Fingers to Fists: Introductory Course. The Arse Class: version 2.3.*

Terrence Higgins Trust Publications: *The Bottom Line*, Second Edition, 2004, Code 124. The Manual, Third Edition, 2005, Code 287.

Chapter Nine: Let's Talk About Sex

1) Sigma: *Time for more: findings from the National Gay Men's Sex Survey, 2000*. Sigma Research, 2001 (ISBN 1 872956 62 9). Ref 01C.

2) Sigma: *Know the score: findings from the National Gay Men's Sex Survey, 2001*. Sigma Research, 2002 (ISBN 1 872956 64 5). Ref 02D.

3) Sigma: *Out and about: findings from the United Kingdom Gay Men's Sex Survey, 2002*. Sigma Research, 2003 (ISBN 1 872956 71 8). Ref 03F.

4) Sigma: *On the move: findings from the United Kingdom Gay Men's Sex Survey, 2003*. Sigma Research, 2004 (ISBN 1 872956 77 7). Ref 04G.

5) Sigma: *Risk and reflexion: findings from the United Kingdom Gay Men's Sex Survey, 2004.* Sigma Research, 2005 (ISBN 1 872956 81 5). Ref 05C.

6) Sigma: *Time for more: findings from the National Gay Men's Sex Survey, 2000.* Sigma Research, 2001 (ISBN 1 872956 62 9). Ref 01C.

7) Elford, J., Bolding, G., Sherr, L. and Hart, G. *Trends in sexual behaviour among London homosexual men 1998–2003: implications for HIV prevention and sexual health promotion.* Sex Transm Infect. 2004 Dec;80(6):451–4. City University, Institute of Health Sciences, St Bartholomew School of Nursing and Midwifery, 24 Chiswell Street, London EC1Y 4TY, UK.

8) Elford, J., Bolding G., Sherr, L., Hart, G. *High risk sexual behaviour among London gay men: no longer increasing.* AIDS 2005, 19: 2171–2174, City University London, Institute of Health Sciences, St Bartholomew School of Nursing and Midwifery, London, UK.

Chapter Ten: The Nuts, Bolts (and Screws) of Sex

1) Stall, R., Paul, J. P. et al. *Alcohol use, drug use and alcohol-related problems among men who have sex with men: the Urban Men's Health Study.* Addiction. 2001 Nov;96(11):1589–601. PMID: 11784456 [PubMed – indexed for MEDLINE]. Division of HIV/AIDS Prevention, Behavioural Intervention Research Branch, Centers for Disease Control and Prevention, Atlanta, Georgia 30333, USA.

Part IV: Sex Problems

Chapter Thirteen: Sexually Transmitted Infections

1) Dodds, J. and Mersey, D. *Sexual Health Survey of Gay Men, London 2004, Annual Summary Report.* Royal Free and University College Medical School, Department of Primary Care and Populations Sciences, Centre for Sexual Health and HIV Research.

2, 3) Health Protection Agency (HPA). Data from *Mapping the Issues: HIV and other Sexually Transmitted Infections in the United Kingdom*: 2005 available at http://www.hpa.org.uk/hpa/publications/hiv_sti_2005/default.htm.

4, 5) Sigma: *Risk and reflexion: findings from the United Kingdom Gay Men's Sex Survey, 2004.* Sigma Research, 2005 (ISBN 1 872956 81 5). Ref 05C.

6, 7, 8, 9) Health Protection Agency (HPA). Data from *Mapping the Issues: HIV and other Sexually Transmitted Infections in the United Kingdom*: 2005 available at http://www.hpa.org.uk/hpa/publications/hiv_sti_2005/default.htm.

10) Sigma: *Risk and reflexion: findings from the United Kingdom Gay Men's Sex Survey, 2004.* Sigma Research, 2005 (ISBN 1 872956 81 5). Ref 05C.

11) Goh, B. 'Sexually Transmitted Infections', Journal of STI's. 2005 vol 81: 448–452.

12) Katz, M. et al. *Post-exposure treatment of people exposed to the human immunodeficiency virus through sexual contact or injection drug use.* NEJM 336:1097–1100,1997.

Chapter Fourteen: Penis Problems

1) Feldman, H. A., Goldstein, I., Dimitrios, G.H. et al. *Impotence and its medical and psychosocial correlates: results of the Massachusetts male aging study.* J Urol 1994;151:54–61.

Chapter Fifteen: Testicular Problems

1) Dearnaley, D. P., Huddart, R. A. and Horwich, A. *Managing testicular cancer.* BMJ 2001;322:1583–1588. Academic Unit of Clinical Oncology, Royal Marsden NHS Trust, Sutton SM2 5PT.

REFERENCES

Chapter Seventeen: Sex Addiction

1) Sigma: *Risk and reflexion: findings from the United Kingdom Gay Men's Sex Survey, 2004*. Sigma Research, 2005 (ISBN 1 872956 81 5). Ref 05C.

2) Bolding, G., Davis, M. et al. *Use of gay Internet sites and views about on-line health promotion among men who have sex with men*. AIDS Care. 2004 Nov;16 (8):993–1001. City University London, Institute of Health Sciences, St Bartholomew School of Nursing and Midwifery, London.

Chapter Eighteen: Drugs: Safer Use and Addiction

1) Sigma: *Vital Statistics: Gay Men's Sex Survey, 2005*. Sigma Research, 2005 (www.sigmaresearch. org.uk/data05/All_England_2005.pdf).

2) Sigma: *Risk and reflexion: findings from the United Kingdom Gay Men's Sex Survey, 2004*. Sigma Research, 2005 (ISBN 1 872956 81 5). Ref 05C.

Chapter Nineteen: Drugs, Health and Sex

1, 2) Bolding, G., Sherr, L. and Elford, J. *Use of anabolic steroids and associated health risks among gay men attending London gyms*. Addiction 2002 Feb 97 (2) 195–203. Department of Primary Care and Population Sciences and Royal Free Centre for HIV Medicine, Royal Free and University College Medical School, University College London, Royal Free Campus, London, UK.

3) Ryan, H., Wortley, P. M. et al. *Smoking among lesbians, gays, and bisexuals: a review of the literature*. Am J Prev Med. 2001 Aug;21(2):142–9. Office on Smoking and Health, Centers for Disease Control and Prevention, Atlanta, Georgia 30341–3717, USA.

INDEX